D0079949

# Important Notice

The information in this book is designed to provide health information for the purposes of reference and guidance and to accompany, not replace, the services of a qualified healthcare practitioner or physician. It is not the intent of the authors or the publisher to recommend or prescribe any substance to cure, mitigate, treat, or prevent any disease. None of the statements in this book have been evaluated by the Food and Drug Administration. In the event you use this information with or without seeking medical attention, the authors and publisher shall not be liable or otherwise responsible for any loss, damage, or injury caused or arising out of, directly or indirectly, by the information contained in this book or its use.

# Healing Across Cultures & The Good Life

An Approach To Holistic Health

Todd Pesek, M.D. | Ronald Reminick, Ph.D. | Murali Nair, Ph.D.

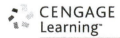
CENGAGE
Learning™

Australia • Brazil • Japan • Korea • Mexico • Singapore • Spain • United Kingdom • United States

# CENGAGE
## Learning™

**Healing Across Cultures & The
Good Life: An Approach To Holistic Health
Todd Pesek, M.D. I Ronald Reminick, Ph.D. I
Murali Nair, Ph.D.**

ALL RIGHTS RESERVED. No part of this work covered by the copyright herein be reproduced, transmitted, stored or used in any form or by any means graphic, electronic, or mechanical, including but not limited to recording, scanning, digitizing, taping, Web distribution, information networks, or information storage and retrieval systems, except as permitted under Section 107 or 108 of the 1976 United States Copyright Act, without the prior written permission of the authors.

For product information and technology assistance, contact us at
**Cengage Learning Customer & Sales Support, 1-800-354-9706**

For permission to use material from this text or product,
submit all requests online at **cengage.com/permissions**
Further permissions questions can be emailed to
**permissionrequest@cengage.com**

Executive Editors:
 Maureen Staudt
 Michael Stranz

Senior Project Development Manager:
 Linda deStefano

Marketing Specialist:
 Courtney Sheldon

Senior Production/Manufacturing Manager:
 Donna M. Brown

PreMedia Manager:
 Joel Brennecke

Sr. Rights Acquisition Account Manager:

 Todd Osborne

Cover Image:
Todd Pesek, M.D. I Ronald Reminick, Ph.D. I
Murali Nair, Ph.D.

**Compilation © 2010 Cengage Learning**

ISBN-13: 978-1-111-22287-1

ISBN-10: 1-111-22287-8

**Cengage Learning**
5191 Natorp Boulevard
Mason, Ohio 45040
USA

Cengage Learning is a leading provider of customized learning solutions with office locations around the globe, including Singapore, the United Kingdom, Australia, Mexico, Brazil, and Japan. Locate your local office at:
**international.cengage.com/region.**

Cengage Learning products are represented in Canada by Nelson Education, Ltd.
For your lifelong learning solutions, visit **custom.cengage.com.**
Visit our corporate website at **cengage.com.**

Printed in the United States of America

# Dedications

We offer this work with unbounded love to all our cosmic family. We are all brothers and sisters every last being, we are all one. We honor the interconnectedness of us all. Above all, however, we dedicate this work to our children. All of our children, for it is from them who we have borrowed the land, sky, water and air. We must return these beings in all their beautiful, mystical majesty. And, to you for receiving this humble offering with an open heart.

To my wife, Leah, and to my daughters, Kaia and Lily. With infinite love and reverence! And, to my elders, who selflessly give of their knowledge and wisdom.

**Todd**

To my wife, Wendy Collura, who has been an essential sounding board for our work on this book.

**Ron**

To my centenarian friends from different cultures who have shared freely their secrets of long life with me.

**Murali**

# Acknowledgements

This work was supported by the Center for Healing Across Cultures, the Graduate College, the College of Liberal Arts and Social Sciences, and the College of Science, Cleveland State University, Cleveland, Ohio, U.S.

The authors wish to thank their many supporters, without whose help this work would not have been possible, from our families and friends to the people of the varied countries in which we work. You are too numerous to mention, but we know who you are and you know who you are. We are particularly indebted to the healers and elders, our guides — the keepers of this treasure trove of knowledge and wisdom. We whole-heartedly express our gratitude to you all for so willingly and forthrightly giving your time and attention to teach us about your professions, practices, beliefs and wisdom. And, many, many thanks for the continued welcome for further research and collaboration toward sustainable, global holistic health promotion through traditional health and wellness practices.

Lastly, we would like to express our sincere thanks to our publishing group and our peer reviewers whose careful attention to detail and critical reviews make this a much stronger work.

**Todd Pesek, M.D.** is a private practice physician in Northeastern Ohio where he specializes in preventive, integrative, holistic medicine. He is a Health Sciences Professor at Cleveland State University, Cleveland, Ohio where he teaches, researches and serves including as Director of the Center for Healing Across Cultures.

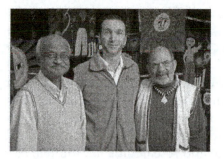

Authors in the Center for Healing Across Cultures, Cleveland State University, Cleveland, Ohio, U.S. From left to right, Professor Murali Nair, Ph.D., Professor Todd Pesek, M.D., and Professor Ron Reminick, Ph.D. In the background is a Maya tapestry. Photograph by Don Bensman Photography.

Dr. Todd received his medical doctorate from The Ohio State University College of Medicine and the Cleveland Clinic, Cleveland, Ohio. He completed his training in Medicine at Case Western Reserve University School of Medicine, St. Vincent Charity Hospital, Cleveland, Ohio.

Raised in the mountains of Appalachia in rural Pennsylvania, he has embraced his calling of holistic health and wellness from an early age. His passion and purpose began with childhood rambles in those very woods, gathering comfort and learning truths from his elders and from nature, and have blossomed into extensive study and collaboration with traditional healers and preventive, integrative, holistic practitioners worldwide. So inspired, Dr. Todd has dedicated himself to the pursuit of keeping people healthy through the tenets of hydration, whole foods nutrition, alkalinization, and detoxification and by an immersion into the healing plants and traditional practices of his own Appalachian tradition, as well as healing plants and practices of other cultures and practitioners learned on his journey.

His work sheds light on holistic health and wellness via deep healing traditions, how they have helped us maintain deep personal health and wellness, and, most importantly, how they can help us stay healthy and filled with vitality in sustainable fashion now.

At Cleveland State University, he teaches Healing Across Cultures, Culture and Health, Environmental Health, and Complementary and Alternative Medicine, where he integrates his international research and scholarship findings in preventive, integrative, holistic health and the secrets of long life as he extends his classroom walls to sacred spaces worldwide.

Dr. Todd has authored numerous publications, documentaries, and academic models in preventive, integrative, holistic health and wellness, and sustainability. He is an internationally prominent speaker with engaging messages who makes his home in rural Northeastern Ohio, where he continues to ramble through the woods to gain inspiration and be renewed by the Earth and Cosmos.

**Ron Reminick, Ph.D.** is an Anthropology Professor, and, Co-Director, Center for Healing Across Cultures, Cleveland State University.

He is a psychological anthropologist who earned his doctorate in Anthropology from the University of Chicago in 1973. He has been studying about and researching in Ethiopia, Africa for the last 42 years. His original fieldwork in Ethiopia (late 1960's) focused on gender identity, ritual symbolism, and traditional health and wellness practices. Dr. Reminick is one of very few three time Fulbright Scholars in the world. His Fulbright tenure has been in Ethiopia throughout. These awards allowed him to contribute to the establishment of a Master's Program in Anthropology at Addis Abeba University, a social sciences curriculum at Bahir Dar University, and supervise a number of groundbreaking ethnographic research projects regionally.

In addition to numerous transformational scholarly articles written on gender identity, ritual symbolism and traditional health and wellness practices, Dr. Ron has also published a theoretical book on ethnicity, a book on African-American ethnicity, a book on the evolution of Addis Abeba, the capital city of Ethiopia, and has co-edited a book, with Drs. Pesek and Nair, on the Healing Traditions of India. At present Dr. Ron teaches courses on Ethiopia, Healing Across Cultures, and Psychological Anthropology, and he continues to research health and healing throughout the world.

**Murali Nair, Ph.D.** is a Social Work Professor, Director of the India Experience Program, and Co-Director, Center for Healing Across Cultures, Cleveland State University.

He received his Doctorate in Social Welfare from Columbia University in New York. For the past thirty years he has been involved in conducting field research on traditional healing practices in Kerala, the southwestern corner of India. He conducts study abroad, full emersion programs in India for diverse students, faculty and helping professionals. Dr. Nair is a Fulbright Scholar to Sri Lanka where he studied traditional healing and secrets of long life. Dr. Nair has been working with centenarians on the secrets of long life and health and wellness for decades. Dr. Nair also specializes in microenterprise for sustainability and health promotion internationally.

At Cleveland State University he teaches courses on Healing Across Cultures, Asian Americans and Alternative Health Systems. He has written several books, including The Art of Community Service: Volunteering and Service Learning -3rd edition (Co-author), Macro Practice: A Generalist Approach – 8th edition (Co-author), Genius in Public Housing: Writings of the Residents – 2nd edition (Editor), Issues in Canadian Human Services (Co-editor), and Healing Traditions of India (Co-editor). Dr. Nair is on the Editorial Board and is the Book Review Editor of the Journal of Baccalaureate Social Work.

# Contents

Dedication

Acknowledgements

Foreword by Warren Grossman, Ph.D.

**Part 1: Learning from Traditions**

**Part 2: Interconnectedness**

**Part 3: Secrets of Long Life**

# Foreword

This meaningful book is for the reader who wants a healthy balance in their life. It explores a framework for enjoying striving toward a better existence. It provides a holistic perspective, practical knowledge, and even wisdom from ancient traditions. It also adds scientific findings from recent research in support of these ancient ways.

The authors combine their expertise in scientific research regarding longevity and time-honored ways to achieve health and wellness. These are practiced in traditional indigenous cultures, including the people of the Americas, India, and parts of Africa. They present their findings in the context of modern day life, and suggest how to apply this wisdom.

You might find yourself asking, "What is a good life? How can I become more whole? By what paths can I achieve health and wellness — biologically, psychologically, and spiritually? How can I transcend our culture of popular media and corporate profit motives?" This book addresses these questions and even more.

The authors believe that we are all connected in a global ecosystem that exerts a deep influence on our lives. The interconnectedness of mind, body, spirit, and environment must not be ignored.

They explain the notions of environment, body, mind, and spirit, and their influence on health. The authors refer to this complex system of relationships as the "ecosystem of health". This is served through a set of straightforward practices rooted in tradition. These methods of achieving health and wellness are grounded in nature. They provide a path to happiness, peace of mind, and a deeper sense of self.

As you read this book, you will encounter ideas about living well, being healthy, and personal growth, through balance and connection to nature. These ideas are not merely limited to the Western orientation of reducing symptoms by way of allopathic medicine. Many of these principles emerge from ancient cultures, whose traditions allowed growth, and even wisdom.

Why should you study this book? Because it will help you to become more intellectually courageous, as you face the universal challenges of hope, becoming, and fulfillment.

Cleveland, Ohio

May 2010

Warren Grossman, Ph.D.

Healer and Author, *To be Healed by the Earth* and *Earth/Heart*

# Chapter 1
# Healing Across Cultures:
# A Repository of Knowledge

*"Knowledge has three degrees-opinion, science, illumination. The means or instrument of the first is sense; of the second, dialectic; of the third, intuition."*

**Plotinus**

*"All truth passes through three stages: first, it is ridiculed; second, it is violently opposed; and third, it is accepted as self-evident."*

**Arthur Schopenhauer**

*"To myself I am only a child playing on the beach, while vast oceans of truth lie undiscovered before me."*

**Sir Isaac Newton**

To appreciate and strive toward the Good Life we can learn from the traditions that have sustained humanity for millennia. These traditions, kept alive in cultures throughout the world, offer us answers to questions of survivability, *joi de vivre*, cultural and spiritual development. There is a new wave of reformation building in cultures around the world. In the U.S. it is recognized as "New Age" and rides the crest of the information revolution we are now experiencing. It harkens back to traditional practices supplanted by cosmocentric worldviews, practices that offer the promise of fulfillment, health, and environmental sustainability. Shamanism, yoga, Taoism, nutritional information from tradition and science, ancient therapeutic techniques that modern medicine is rediscovering to great advantage, traditional introspective techniques that open portals to personal understanding and deep appreciation of our cosmos, to mention a few, all provide paths to the Good Life. In a time of turmoil, conflict, fear, confusion about global affairs, anxiety about the meaning of life, our deliverance can be achieved through grounding via nature and the rich resources of tradition by which humanity has thrived.

We offer this book to provide knowledge about holistic health and maintaining personal and community vitality through an appreciation of the traditions and ancient practices of cultures around the world. Our perspectives are drawn from our experiences leading up to and including decades of field studies and experience the word over. We are a 21st century holistic medical doctor and ethnobotanist who works predominantly in the Great Lakes and Appalachian regions of North America, the Maya Mountains of Central America, and Amazonian and Andean highlands of South America; a three time Fulbright award-winning psychological anthropologist whose major work is in Ethiopia; and a Fulbright Scholar and Professor of social work who has accomplished important studies in India and Sri Lanka. Together we direct Cleveland State University's Center for Healing Across Cultures founded to facilitate positive change in health, wellness and sustainability through the research and application of traditional modalities for the maintenance of health and wellness, heightening of consciousness, happiness, and wisdom in the pursuit of healthier people, their communities, and our living environment. For our efforts, we have recently been awarded the United States Presidential Award for Volunteer Service.

Our perspective holds that we are all inextricably connected in a global ecosystem with tethers to the cosmos and that the influences on our lives reach deeply into the molecular processes of life and outwardly to/from the cosmic forces all of which we are still in the process of discovering.

 The process of scientific and intuitive discovery brings with it a personal, community, national, and global responsibility to commit ourselves to nurture a healthy planet and to expose those who violate the principles of nature, principles that have maintained life for billions of years. Modern science and medicine, from physics and molecular biology to anthropology and philosophy, have laid the groundwork for reaffirming the wisdom of traditions and for the appreciation of the awesome complexity of living systems and life forms with whom we are in community.

In this book, we describe and explain what we mean by "environment", "body", "mind", and "spirit" all of which are interconnected and influence our ways of being. This interconnectedness, this incredibly complex system of relationships, we refer to as the "ecosystem of health" and it involves the holistic perspectives which we delve into in the chapters following. It provides for us a path to greater health and happiness, peace of mind, appreciation of nature, a deep sense of self and the meaning of life, and a sense of fulfillment — the Good Life.

It is our position that medicine and healing are not synonymous, nor should healing be the application of a drug prescribed by a medical doctor to treat disease. A note on the meaning of medicine: The father of modern medicine, Hippocrates, who lived twenty-four hundred years ago in ancient Greece declared that education and food are the greatest medicine. As he pointed out then, knowledge is the path to a greater consciousness and at least a part of this health knowledge involves food, and, as we know today, its phytochemicals including plant sterols, pigments, antioxidants, vitamins, minerals, enzymes, and cofactors among others. This is closer to healing.

In this book we address the knowledge we have gained about the survival and evolution of life and living communities over past millennia. This knowledge exists at the cognitive, emotional as well as pragmatic levels. It is fairly easy to understand how ideas, reason, and technology are important applications of knowledge, but more difficult to understand what emotional intelligence is and how it works, yet it is a very important aspect of wellness and the maintenance of vitality throughout life. One aspect of this book, therefore, is to point out what this is and how to develop it.

The major purpose of this book, however, is to demonstrate the importance of a holistic perspective in creating a more viable way of healthful living and the Good Life. This perspective sees the flora, fauna, and all the earthly substances of our planet as interconnected in an imperfect but, when uninterrupted, self-correcting balance of evolving phenomena. Natural systems function in a harmonious balance, a sort of give-take equilibrium. Dysfunction and imbalance open an organism and the system to disease and death. Because we live on a planet of awesome diversity, we have the responsibility to discover and understand the basis of this diversity in order to preserve, rather than destroy, the resources by which we live. We have the responsibility to know what threatens the wellness of all living things and to eliminate these threats from our lives. We have the responsibility to know what contributes to our wellness, of organisms and communities, and to preserve and value these.

Other purposes of this book are: to show that traditional healing systems offer valuable information for modern persons and communities; guidance toward the development of both provider-based and individual holistic health and wellness ideals to be used in health maintenance; and to provide a health model for individuals in shaping their strategies for wellness.

The idea that wellness requires balance among the elements of mind, body, and spirit within an environmental context is evident throughout the thoughts, beliefs, and practices of traditional healers as well as in those of holistic healthcare professionals. This holistic paradigm expresses universal themes found in many, if not most, cultures of the world emphasizing balance, respect, and care for a sustainable environment. This book concisely conceptualizes the vast and growing sea of information on health and wellness that is becoming un-navigable and often misleading. A return to the basics or a "return to our roots" is warranted. An increasing number of professionals and laypersons are hungry for more information and guidance regarding the multi-dimensional field of culturally grounded holistic health.

There are two major movements in medicine today. Consider them as two very different approaches toward health. Conventional medicine, for the most part, deals with disease and the application of drugs supplied by the pharmaceutical industry, to the treatment of disease. The other rapidly growing movement, incorporating traditional practices, is recognized today as Complementary and Alternative Medicine (CAM) and treats afflictions with naturally occurring resources and traditional practices as has been our practice throughout humanity save the last few hundred years. CAM is broadly defined by the National Institutes of Health (NIH) as "a group of diverse medical and health care systems, practices, and products that are not generally considered part of conventional medicine." NIH established the Center for Complementary and Alternative Medicine (NCCAM) to "explore complementary and alternative healing practices in the context of rigorous science, train CAM researchers, and disseminate authoritative information to the public and professionals."

The recognition of the efficacy of this approach by the general population and the marketing of natural products such as vitamins and other nutritional supplements is growing exponentially as the conventional model of healthcare, more accurately seen as "disease-care" breaks down logistically and economically. The wave of this revolution rests on the prevention of disease and the maintenance of vitality through the access of naturally occurring resources and the knowledge gleaned from both ancient traditions and modern science. Along with this recent cultural consciousness is the growing awareness of the serious toxic overload we have created in our environment and the serious illnesses that have been the result. The often economically debilitating high cost of pharmaceuticals and the serious side effects of these drugs have also influenced a growing number of knowledgeable individuals to change their lifestyle and enjoy greater health and vitality. Holistic medicine promises to shape an economically viable system of health maintenance through education and by broadcasting information about the ever-present toxins that pollute our bodies, minds, and our environment. A cursory survey of magazines, books, news articles, the proliferation of nutritional supplement businesses and studios of yoga, tai chi, pilates, massage therapy, gyms, spas, and health clubs, to name a few, all attest to this movement of individuals taking responsibility for the quality of their lives.

Evidence of ancient civilization and its views into the nature of health and wellness is prevalent in contemporary cultures the world over. Indian scholars, for example, six thousand years ago, were evolving the art of healing—many of these practices continue today. In many of their ancient writings, healers communicated the ways of healing a person's body, mind, and spirit. For example, the *Charaka Samhita* is believed to have arisen around 2,400-2,200 years ago. It is thought to be one of the oldest and the most important ancient codified authoritative writings on Ayurveda healing, which is also a practiced way of life.

Indigenous peoples the world over believe that entities in this world, including plants, insects, birds, animals, and human beings, possess an innate ability to heal themselves without external intervention. It seems plausible that if the body can heal itself from a wound or a broken bone, then it could heal itself from cancer and other grave ailments. Clear evidence of this is consistently found in medical records.

In modern society, there is an ever-growing disconnection from the natural world. This is worrisome because we are a constituent in nature and as such are inextricably interconnected with and dependent upon nature for our wellbeing.

A careful study of natural phenomena reveals harmony and the integration of life forms. For example, certain botanicals produce a kind of olfactory indicator that allures or distracts insects, birds and animals, thus informing them on what to eat and what not to eat at certain times. This instinct sustains their life. It is not only from animals' interactions with plants by which we may learn from nature, but also from careful observation of the plants themselves, their modes of adaptation and growth. Through mindful interaction, nature also teaches us how to keep fit. For example, from housecats to lions on the Serengeti, felines always stretch in different poses as part of their daily routine—not only felines however, but dogs too and, in fact, all animals need stretching in their lives. A classic yoga pose for rest and rejuvenation is the "downward facing dog" where one stretches on all four limbs with the pelvis high in the air. We now know that by doing so not only contributes to our mobility and flexibility, but it also improves our circulation and lymphatic flow; something essential to us all.

Since time immemorial, people have enhanced their own health, living in balance with nature, engaging in physical and mental exercise, and by eating well. Healers the world over have taught our inevitable connection to nature and nature's timeless nurturance of humankind. In ancient times, people learned from and worshipped nature: earth and the cosmos. Spirituality and healing have always been combined in tradition. Even today in Indic lifeways, Taoist and other eastern philosophies, Native American and Appalachian cultures, and traditionally living indigenous peoples the world over, nature worship in spirituality is uniformly present. Oral traditions of healing often have thousands of years of history, and, over the years, have brought to the forefront some of the prominent healing techniques of today. Some Eastern traditions can appreciate noble lineages in different forms of healing reaching back millennia. These belief systems and practices are passed on from one generation to another. It is unfortunate in Western society that many in the scientific community negate the oral traditions and ask for proof. Only very recently, in the U.S., the writings of Deepak Chopra[1] and others brought attention to the public of the importance of ancient India's healing traditions. A 2nd century B.C. Indian physician, Caraka, systematically outlined different subjects: embryology, human anatomy, digestive system, circulatory system, respiration, brain function, pharmacology, and other practices of medicine. Caraka Samhita[2], the writings of Caraka, even now are considered among the oldest, most ancient and important authoritative writings on the aforementioned Ayurveda.[3] In 1898, a Caraka club was formed in New York to propagate his form of ancient healing in the United States.[4] The Indian healing practices of Ayurveda and astrological methods go back millennia.[3] The Ayurvedic form of healing enriches the qualities of life of a person through the different sensations of sound, touch, vision, taste, smell, position, and astral intuition. Recent popular publications like the Encyclopedia of Healing Therapies [5], the Encyclopedia of Natural Medicine[6], and Oriental Medicine: Ancient Arts of Healing[4], contain hundreds of references to Indian and Chinese traditional healing practices. Much like the Appalachian mountain peoples, Native Americans and others who embrace environmental stewardship, the cosmocentric worldviews and recognition of the elements of nature are very much incorporated into the healing practices of traditional people the world over.

There is much value in the understanding of healing traditions, as well as lessons for how we as a society can survive in harmony with nature. Natural and herbal health/healing practices have been developed by traditional healers through careful observation and consistently refined trial and error—in effect the scientific method. These practices have been used successfully and passed down from generation to generation via oral and written traditions as texts and stories of health and wellness. We recognize that the gold standard in medicine, for the evaluation of a pharmaceutical intervention, is the randomized double blind clinical trial. It is our position that although this is one good tool, we should also recognize that traditional medicine, practiced by indigenous peoples since the dawn of humanity, has been based on observation and testing over long periods of time, discovering what plant medicines work and what plants do not and what plants are toxic to humans. The process of the search, the discovery, the use, the testing by trial and error, and the establishment of the particular plant in the technology of the culture is not that far removed from what modern scientists do today, which is to discover what already exists, report it, communicate it to a wider audience, and test its efficacy. Clinical trials of well-designed observational studies, with either a cohort or a case–control design, are just as reliable as compared with those in randomized, controlled trials on the same topic.[7] The "practice" of clinical medicine is essentially an experiment on an *n* of one, the patient. Everyone is different, however. Traditional practices as learned through generations of shared learning with our natural world warrant serious examination because they represent millennia of observational clinical trials culminating in traditional practices. This knowledge must not be lost with the passing of the older generations. Younger generations must be encouraged to take an interest in and see psychological and material rewards from learning the folk medical and healing practices of those aging family members still alive and able to share their knowledge. This traditional intergenerational interaction can diffuse into modern urban society and further inspire many younger and middle aged individuals today who, in ever increasing numbers, believe in the extensive benefits of CAM. For decades, modern medicine has been not only skeptical of but often closed off to the knowledge and effectiveness of various forms of alternative medicine. A range of medical and health traditions of indigenous North America, the Appalachian Mountains, the rainforests of Central and South America, Africa, east Asia, and, very importantly, India, continue to be used by those who embrace their preventive and curative benefits.

Global health and wellness is greatly facilitated by traditional healing. More than 80% of the worlds population relies on traditional healing for primary healthcare[8,9] and greater than 25% of modern medical drugs stem from traditional healing knowledge.[8,9] Indeed, there is heavy reliance on CAM practitioners within Western cultures.[10] Interestingly, Dr. David Eisenberg's published and widely circulated findings on the prevalence of CAM usage[10] was initially met with substantial skepticism and even overt criticism. Now, over a decade later, his numbers have been confirmed by NIH surveys.[11] In December of 2008, NCCAM along with the National Center for Health Statistics (an entity within the Centers for Disease Control and Prevention) released new findings on CAM use in the U.S. The findings are developed from the "National Health Interview Survey 2007", an annual survey of Americans regarding their health and illness- related experiences and practices. The CAM component gathered information from 23,393 adults aged 18 years or older as well as 9,417 children aged 17 years and under. Essentially, it demonstrates that approximately 38 % adults and approximately 12 % of children use CAM.[11] Interesting, that medical science is beginning to recognize what traditions have known for generations. It is time that we listen closely.

We propose a holistic collaboration that combines modern medical science with traditional healers and traditional healing practices around the world.[12] We believe that this holistic integrative approach to health knowledge will provide not only ways of healing ourselves without the side effects of pharmacology, but a reawakening to the benefits and health-giving resources of nature's bounty. From this will emerge a respect for maintaining the environment that nurtures the world: people, animals, and plants. The growing realization of the intricate connections among mind, body, and spirit in the context of our natural world is long overdue in modern society. Our understanding of Healing Across Cultures sets us on a path that can lead only to a better sense of self within the context of the cosmos—a more and more appropriate idea as we increasingly discover ourselves as a global community. We are returning home to the age old lessons of health, wellness, and survival within nature that have existed since time immemorial.

Our ancestors were terribly aware of their vulnerability to the natural environment and those other groups who threatened their stability. This situation motivated certain individuals to develop a technology in their attempt to stabilize their health and their social solidarity. This technology has diffused to contemporary generations and survives in various modalities in those individuals who are the cultural reservoirs of their healing traditions.[12] These healers and shamans realize that social process influences the health and well being of their people. In primitive cultures the approach to life is integral with the environment and conservative with its natural resources. It is appreciated by indigenous peoples that wasteful practices are antithetical to survival since no one wants to destroy what is depended upon.

Indigenous cultures implement much of their values and teachings through ritual, folklore and other traditional knowledge including traditional botanical knowledge and traditional healing knowledge. This approach is a strong influence in the socialization of the young who live and teach these healing traditions to ensuing generations. Indeed, elements of the great healing traditions are beginning to contribute to the amelioration of many of our modern day diseases including illnesses that result from lifestyle. And, the burgeoning of the CAM industry based on traditional phytomedicines is largely consumer driven.[13]

We are learning from these traditions and traditional healing practices and are applying them to modern day health problems. Together, science and tradition can maintain modalities for sustainability and more harmonious coexistence with our natural world. With the knowledge of science and the wisdom of ancient tradition we can find our way to a growing global consciousness and a healthful sustainable environment.

# Chapter 2
# Environment: Nurturer of Us All

*"There is a thing, formless yet complete. Before heaven and earth it existed. Without sound, without substance, it stands alone and unchanging. It is all pervading and unfailing. We do not know its name, but we call it Tao. Being one with nature, the sage is in accord with the Tao."*

**Lao Tzu**

*"Whenever we try to pick out anything by itself, we find it hitched to everything else in the universe."*

**John Muir**

*"Our task must be to free ourselves by widening our circle of compassion to embrace all living creatures and the whole of nature and its beauty."*

**Albert Einstein**

**Our Cosmic Connections, Birthing and Beyond: We are but stellar dust**

Astronomical physics tells us that the universe, as we know it, came into being with the "Big Bang." The Big Bang generally refers to the concept that the universe is rapidly expanding from an exceedingly small, hot, dense initial condition at some finite time roughly 14 billion years ago. It also tells that the universe continues to expand at an accelerating rate to this day.[1]

There are a variety of theories as to what occurred just prior to the Big Bang, however, we do not know what preceded it. Theory has it that the universe exploded out in a matter of milliseconds! We do not know the state of the universe at the moment of the Big Bang. Nor do we know what "banged." For simplicity, we refer to the universe as everything to which we are physically connected, including us. That's correct! One might say we, the universe, created ourselves to learn about us!

The universe includes, among other cosmic bodies: planet Earth and her moon; the solar system within which we are situated. Our galaxy, the Milky Way, which is our galaxy; and the billions of galaxies that exist in our known universe. The Milky Way is a spiral type galaxy, and, our familiar sun is one of about 200-

400 billion stars in the Milky Way[2]. There are perhaps 500 billion other galaxies, some of which are as large as trillions of stars. Recent astronomical findings suggest that we may know only ¼ of what the universe is! The universe also contains (or does it?) "dark matter" and "dark energy."[1]

We understand very little about dark matter and dark energy. Basically, these are presumed based on gravitational realities in our observable universe. Evidently, they make up about three quarters of our universe though and so it is quite interesting that we understand so little about something of such magnitude. We do surmise, however, that they are at least, in part, responsible for the accelerated expansion of our universe.

Gravity is another fundamental force of nature which we know very little about. So, who is to say that dark energy, dark matter, and gravity are not just mere perceptions of something that we have come to observe through an obscured lens? Another way of saying this is that our brain acts as a filter to establish reality as observable reality, this is not actually the case. An extended, but related, aside: what about consciousness? Is it a field like gravity, something we observe and experience, but know very little about? Given the data, it is plausible that consciousness resides outside of us as does gravity.[3] There will be more on this in following chapters. Whatever the case may be, cosmologists, and scientists who study such things the world over have elaborated a number of theories including the existence of parallel universes and multiverses.[1] Generally speaking, the multiverse theory suggests the existence of many more universes just like ours, perhaps with which we interact only through "gravity." Perhaps it is these multiverses which are the dark matter and dark energy.

What does this have to do with our concept of environment? We now know that there are forces out there that influence our lives and impinge, often on a very subtle level, on all living species of our planet.

Our solar system is about two-thirds out of the galactic center of the Milky Way[2] and so when peering into the night sky at the Milky Way stretching across one is peering into the galactic center and when peering into less populated night sky one is peering out into more "empty" space. It's not actually empty though!

Our view of the night sky is constantly changing. It changes in three regular fixed ways with our annual orbit around Earth's sun, our night and day due to the spinning of Earth on her axis, and slightly changing view due to Earths procession (or slight wobbling effect due to the 5 degree tilt in her axis). Our cosmic vista is also changing in irregular ways with the constant expansion of our universe and the disappearance and emergence of stellar bodies. By the way, very little of our universe is actually visible to us given the fact that even our most powerful instruments can only peer into a fraction of its expanse. We really do not know how large it is since we cannot fully see it.

Whether we see it or not, though, we interact with our universe in a multitude of ways we understand and even more ways that we do not understand, but more on this in a bit.

Planet earth came into being, about 4.6 billion years ago, with an accrual of dust and gas or cosmic debris[4,5]. Every atom in our bodies is traceable to this dust and gas as well. Everything in the universe as we know it is comprised of cosmic debris even us!

The Ignition of Life and Our Global Ancestry: We are all brothers and sisters, big and small.

The first life on Earth for which we have evidence is bacteria-like microorganisms found in rocks of western Australia and stromatolites or mats of fossilized microorganisms representing the same time period of about 3.5 billion years ago.[4,5] So we do have a couple of relatively contemporary examples of life on Earth about then, but we do not know if there is anything that predates this, nor do we know if these life forms originated on Earth or, for example, reached Earth in the form of spores or something of the sort from nearby Mars who's history and certain ecological aspects paralleled that of Earth then. Make no mistake, scientists continues to assume that life originated on Earth when it may well not have done so.[4]

Current theories on the "spark" of life, or how early life began, suggest that through the actions of solar and atmospheric energies, lightning and rainfall, various organic molecules formed and accumulated in our oceans. Certain organic molecules have a tendency to aggregate like the oil and vinegar on your favorite salad. These organic molecular aggregations would have been the primeval cell (our greatest grandparent!) which then, through interacting with its environment, began to evolve itself to adapt to its changing environment and vie successfully for what it needed. In doing so, it changed its environment drastically. These early life forms altered the atmospheric conditions of the Earth to a point where other life, first more complex cells, or eukaryotes, became possible, roughly 1.5 billion years ago. Then came multi-cellular organisms about 700 million years ago as well as the first fungi.[4]  There was a lot going on in the oceans.  First chordates appeared in the fossil record about 570 million years ago; then mollusks, jawed fishes and then amphibians appeared on land about 360 million years ago. First evidence of plants is seen about 440 million years ago. Then there were insects and the diversification of land plants shortly thereafter, thanks, in part, to the insects, since they were the major pollinators.  The first dinosaurs and mammals appear about 245 million years ago and so on right up to the earliest evidence of hominids with *Ardipithecus ramidus* about 4.4 million years ago.[4,5]

Our species, *Homo sapiens*, did not evolve until about 200,000 years ago, and we had some competitors of our own. Our distant cousins the Neanderthals, although from a different branch on the hominid tree were from the same progenitor species, *Homo erectus*.  We out-competed our cousins perhaps with our primordial spirit.  In any event, we shared the Earth with another type of humans spawned from our earliest life forms.

An overwhelming scientific and scholarly consensus suggests that all of humanity resided in Africa up until roughly 60,000 years ago.  It was then when our earliest *H. sapien* ancestors, perhaps as few as 150 individuals,[6] began their first trek out of Africa.  This group essentially skirted Asia along the southern seashores and headed for Australia having it settled within a mere 10,000 years. There was then a second wave which moved to populate Asia and India then Europe and Siberia. It was this group which literally disbursed with the four directions approximately 40,000 years ago.  Europe was populated about 30,000 years ago and Siberia was populated approximately 20,000 years ago.  Shortly thereafter, about 12,000 years ago, a group of our hunter-gatherer ancestors traversed the Beringia land bridge from Siberia and moved into the Americas for the first time ever.  It took our resilient, nomadic ancestors roughly 2000 years thenceforth to span the entire longitude of North, Central and South America and there you have it, we had settled the entire planet within essentially 50,000 years of traveling.[6]

Science has indeed shown what great thinkers have professed for millennia — we are all literally brothers and sisters, indeed cut from the same energetic tapestry which embodies humanity.  These thousands of generations experienced and learned from preceding generations whose accumulated experience was codified in language and communicated to future generations.  Early peoples would observe and interact with their surroundings, grow to understand what intellectual and material technology they would need to adapt and survive and proceed with their lifeways. Learning through experience and discovering what already exists is a primary tenet of science. For example, this tree sap is red, I wonder if it treats the blood, or this root is yellow perhaps it is good for the liver. If they then work after being tested on humans in these intuited capacities they kept it, if it did not, they discarded it and so evolved the traditional pharmacopoeia born of generations of shared learning.

In a very general sense, we can conceptualize our environment within a holistic perspective as a configuration of highly interconnected material and nonmaterial things acting under certain conditions that influence the surrounding reach of its forces in a given moment. In a less general sense we can identify air, water, minerals, and organisms that influence life forms on this planet. We also include intangible, invisible influences such as sound, temperature, nuances of light, microscopic and submicroscopic organisms, pollutions of air, water, food and animals, ultraviolet and electromagnetic radiation, chemical reactions, subtle influences of the sun and moon, gravity, repetitive patterns of sight and sound that either deaden or enlighten the mind, and the merging of the forces of emotional energy between two or more organisms in attraction or repulsion in love or its antithesis.

The understanding and appreciation of the particular elements of our environment at the various levels of action will empower human beings to recognize that which is inimical to health and wellness and to foster those elements that elevate wellness and consciousness of the individual which will in turn create a community of human beings that will contribute to the powerful forces of potentiation that reside within us all.

The remarkable discoveries and advances in science, from molecular biology to astrophysics, has contributed to the capacity for modern human beings to know, understand, and appreciate much of what ancient traditions have intuited for millennia — that we are inextricably intertwined with the natural world and that we need to respect, revere, and care for that which nourishes us.

**Our Environmental Milieu**

Cells are complex membranes surrounding an array of chemical reactions and energetic interactions. These complex reactions and interactions make up cells and have been shaped by millennia of evolution with the natural world. Our cells cluster in communities creating nuclei and foci for specific functions in collaboration. These then give rise to organs that coalesce as an organism. An organism, then, by extension is a community of over a trillion (in humans, 100 trillion) individual cells functioning in relative harmony to maintain balance necessary for life. Since practice makes perfect, we are most well equipped doing what we have done the longest.

The aforementioned sections in chapter two illustrate some very important concepts: our cosmic ancestry; that we are all related; and the immense expanse of time that our evolutionary journey allowed us to become what we are, for better or worse.

This latter point becomes extremely important in answering a number of questions in health today. For example, we have evolved for millennia with sugar and fat in short supply. Our bodies' needs directed us to seek out these nutritive items as they existed in nature. This consumption triggered satiety responses in our brains and nourished our physiology in meeting our needs for caloric and energetic consumption. We would do well in the modern day to mimic these diets low in sugar and fats as it is what our bodies are designed for doing well. We are assaulted with imaging, messaging, and branding toward the contrary, however, with socially irresponsible profit motives contributing to ill health, obesity, diabetes and other diseases of civilization.

Another example is environmental toxicities. Since throughout our evolutionary course we have not been exposed to heavy metals like lead, mercury, cadmium, aluminum, nickel, or plastics like polyvinyl chloride, polystyrene, or polycarbonate/bisphenol A, nor have we been exposed to the multitude of herbicides, pesticides, deicing chemicals, preservatives, dyes, paints, solvents, flame retardants, pharmaceutical drugs, our body does not know how to get rid of these things optimally. What ends up happening, once these toxic materials make their way into our systems, is *sequestration*. The body stores them, normally in fat, away from the vital organs in order to protect organ function. Environmental toxins are quite commonplace now. They are pervasive in our food, water and air. Stuart Lonkey, M.D., a pulmonary and critical care doctor and author of Invisible Killers, cites as many as 200 different toxins which may be found in breast milk! We cannot be healthy in a toxic state and these toxic burdens have become unmanageable through our limited excretory pathways and sequestration of what remains. The alarmingly high rates of cancer in the U.S. is testament to the severe toxic environment we live in. In promotion of health one must both avoid toxins as best as one can, and, one must facilitate excretion of them through detoxification programs.[7] This is discussed further in following chapters.

As a modern population, we have become disconnected from what we have long lived in close connection with—the natural world. Despite this disconnection, we are very much a part of the natural world, and we are dependent upon it. Our intimacy with nature has evolved cultures that have complex cosmocentric perceptions, conceptions, and practices involving our relationship with nature and its gentle exploitation. This contrasts with the capitalistic orientation to nature of exploitation for profit no matter what the consequences. The wisdom and practices of indigenous cultures are encoded in their traditions and kept alive today in spite of the overbearing domination of U.S. individualistic, materialistic, capitalistic, exploitative corporate-ruled society. This ancient wisdom, living with and learning from nature, has lead to the discovery of different types of knowledge that has been passed down generation to generation through predominantly oral traditions. Traditional healing is one such component of this knowledge and holds countless benefits for community health and global health and wellness.[8]

This indigenous knowledge and wisdom that has sustained a balance of nature and a coexistence with other animal and plant species is disappearing as a result of Western acculturation and the loss of the world's sacred natural areas and biodiversities.

Since languages can be taken as a marker of culture and their embedded ancestral wisdom and knowledge, we see that the diversity of languages is rapidly disappearing.[9,10] They are disappearing at an alarming rate. Of the 15,000 languages spoken approximately 70 years ago, there are only 6000 spoken today.[10,11,12] Our planet's natural places and its biodiversity are being lost with the loss of language and culture.

Forests are being lost at a disturbing rate and biodiversity trends illustrate the gravity of the situation we face. The United Nations Food and Agricultural Organization (FAO) determines losses of between 9 million and 12 million hectares (ha, 2.5 acres) per year from 1990 to 2000.[13] FAO further shows that approximately 0.8% of intact forests are being lost on an annual basis and that total yearly rainforest losses range from 5 million to over 20 million ha.[13] Just as forest cover, planetary biodiversity is being lost at a staggering rate as well. According to the Living Planet Index (LPI)[14] which is a marker for biodiversity loss and based on hundreds of vertebrate species in terrestrial, freshwater and marine ecosystems globally, biodiversity is disappearing at alarming rates. During the 30 year interval from 1970-2000, the LPI dropped precipitously by 37% and is indicative of accelerating trends.[14] Global species extinctions are 100-

1000 times that of the natural rate, heralding the 6th mass extinction in the natural history of the earth.[15] Importantly, this mass extinction is precipitated by humans whereas the others were not anthropogenic.

Jeffrey McNeely, chief scientist at International Union for the Conservation of Nature (IUCN), argues that the preservation of indigenous cultural traditions and the tropical forests they live in are inseparable and can only be achieved in concerted fashion. Cultural and biological diversity persist, most notably, in mountainous regions[16] and they must be preserved together. Initiatives focused on culturally ethical sustainable development and conservation of cultural and biological diversity are necessary and can be targeted toward mountainous areas of high cultural and biological diversity with good effect. Traditional healing knowledge and practice is one such potential vehicle for much needed sustainable development.

In dealing with traditional cultural healing knowledge a number of complexities arise with regard to various political agendas, cross-cultural information sharing, intellectual property protection, and benefits sharing.[17,18,19] It seems that historically, no matter how well-intentioned and well negotiated pharmaceutical drug development prospecting has been, the benefits rarely matriculate to communities and/or the holders of the knowledge.[19] There are a number of studies that detail these complexities and offer suggestions on ways to proceed in avoidance of them. Among these studies are several that discuss underlying forces of globalization and make noteworthy submissions for practical procedures in establishing ethical cross-cultural exchange.[20,21] Better still, perhaps as an alternative, less controversial methods and technologies for community benefit should be sought immediately, based on the gravity of our biological and cultural extinction rates.

An alternative that could preclude complex economic and political issues and yet provide potential conservation strategies and support for indigenous communities is the development of traditional healing centers complete with indigenous herbal gardens and the teaching and promoting of indigenous ecological knowledge respect and integration of traditional healing into the respective national healthcare systems.[22] This is based on a phytomedicine model using traditional remedies rather than pharmaceutical drugs in healthcare. Since traditional healers and their healing systems rely more comprehensively on the health of the individual in the context of their healthful environment, communities tended by traditional healers insure a healthy and sustainable ecology.[8]

As an example of this model, we consider the case of the Q'eqchi' Maya of southern Belize where a majority of the population relies on traditional healing for primary healthcare.[22] The Q'eqchi' are one of 20 contemporary Maya cultural groups that have inherited certain environmental and health perceptions from their predecessors who spawned the vast Maya civilization. The importance of environmental respect and sustainability is quite widespread among these extant Maya groups. The Itza Maya of Peten, Guatemala, integrate their food crop cultivation with tropical forest management through various complex species interactions.[23] Their system is maintained by cyclical interaction of indefinite forest regeneration in combination with their sustainable use.[23] The Lacandon Maya of Chiapas, Mexico are rainforest farmers who often cultivate medicinal plants in house gardens, *milpas* (farming plots based on ancient agricultural traditions and which involve cycles in production and rejuvenation of the land), and, secondary milpas (or prior milpas overtaken by the forest in rejuvenation phases), and, they gather wild plants from the jungle.[24] Their practices support the continual regeneration and sustainable use of the rainforest. The Yucatec Maya view the land as a living being that needs to be fed, nurtured and cared for just as us all.[25] The Q'eqchi' Maya of southern Belize have taken a proactive stance in conservation of their healing tradition and their environment for future generations.[22]

## Itzama

*Itzama* (home of the Maya god of wisdom, *Itzamna*, and place of ritual and herbal healing) is a name chosen by members of the Belize Indigenous Training Institute (BITI) and its associated Q'eqchi' Healers Association (QHA) to describe their innovative community-based traditional healing conservation program which is aimed at the preservation of their rainforests and deep cultural traditions through the promotion of traditional healing.[22]

The Q'eqchi' Maya communities of the area lead a traditional lifestyle in this forest and maintain intact traditional medical systems and forest knowledge as part of their culture to this day,[26] their culture has successfully used nature to treat primary and complex ailments and imbalance for thousands of years. In an age when more and more people globally are using viable natural alternatives to conventional medicine, the Maya medical heritage is being documented, recorded, saved and implemented by the Maya themselves as a global model in holistic, sustainable healthcare.

The Itzama project is committed to health promotion, sustainable development, and the conservation of biodiversity and culture through the use of traditional healing systems and rainforest stewardship programs. The elders and traditional healers of the Maya people are leading these programs. They have been implemented in remote villages of rural southern Belize and surrounding areas that are highly dependent on medicinal plants and traditional healing for primary healthcare. And, the model is taking root elsewhere internationally including North America, South America, India and Africa. BITI and the QHA in collaboration with external partners (Inuit Circumpolar Conference, University of Ottawa, Universidad Nacional, Earth Healers and Naturaleza Foundation, and Cleveland State University) have taken the lead in the development of the physical site including the center and gardens, taking plant inventories in the Maya Mountains areas, implementing traditional sustainable plant propagation techniques on site, and developing programming strategies inclusive of protocols for ethical collaboration across cultures. This program holds real promise in enhancing the sustainable management of the medicinal plant resources of the area while enabling local communities to reap health and cultural benefits of the resources without depleting the forests and endangered plant species.

The healers developed the indigenous botanical gardens at the site in order to have a nearby sustainable source of plant material for the treatment of ailments in the villages where they serve as primary care providers. The gardens are also used for healing rites and ceremonies, celebrations of the Maya calendar, demonstrations, educational programming about traditionally used medicinal plants and their conservation, agricultural production for local use by the healers, and local enterprise development.

Given the success of Itzama, it seems appropriate to allow for the promotion of safe, effective traditional healing. The healers can facilitate the dissemination of public health information, provide general front line healthcare as well as first aid and life saving techniques working together with other providers in a concerted educational initiative.

Traditional healing systems are adapted to their respective cultural environments. And particular healers maintain their own ritual and herbal technology derived from their local habitat. Despite this varied assembly of healing traditions and healers—several important themes in healing exist.[8] One of these recurrent themes is that true healing occurs with the support of healthful environmental surroundings. Another is that traditional healers provide sustainable healthcare and have a certain degree of respect for one's environmental surroundings. This is due to their cosmocentric worldviews. Therefore, by advocating for traditional healing, we support healthful environmental surroundings and culturally appropriate conservation of biodiversity and culture.

Perhaps most importantly, these efforts are leading to a more ethical, equitable, sustainable, and efficacious method of healthcare delivery in harmony with the natural world. They could spawn a multitude of mutually beneficial learning engagements between traditional healers and other caregivers internationally that will support the development of healthcare, wellness promotion, and possibilities for the Good Life in a healthy and beautiful environment.

# Chapter 3
# Body: Good Physiology Gives Good Health

*"The vital force is not enclosed in man, but radiates around him like a luminous sphere, and it may be made to act at a distance. In these semi-material rays the imagination of a man may produce healthy or morbid effects."*

**Paracelsus**

*"This we know: the earth does not belong to man, man belongs to the earth. All things are connected like the blood that unites us all. Man did not weave the web of life, he is merely a strand in it. Whatever he does to the web, he does to himself."*

**Chief Seattle**

*"Inconceivable as it seems to ordinary reason - you and all other conscious beings as such - are all in all. Hence this life of yours which you are living is not merely a piece of the entire existence, but is in a certain sense the whole. Thus you can throw yourself flat on the ground, stretched out upon mother earth, with the certain conviction that you are one with her and she with you."*

**Erwin Schroedinger**

We conceive of the body as an energetic organism functioning in an adaptive relationship to its physical, biological, social, cultural, and spiritual environment. The forces of these environments impinge on and influence the organism and that organism feeds back its influence on its diverse environments. This is the perspective of ecology. The organelles of a cell live in the cellular environment. Cells live in the environment of their respective organs, organs live in the environment of the organism. The organism lives within the environment of its five environmental realms and beyond. We note here that sub-cellular study leads one to molecular and even subatomic levels. Subatomic levels once again cast us into the cosmos since we are then dealing with biophotons, electromagnetic radiation and other aspects of our complex nature which we have yet to discover. Suffice it to say that our scientific discoveries have taught us what challenges lay ahead.

Ecology is the scientific study of relationships among the forces that influence an organism and its community and the influences the organism and its community give back. We are all inextricably intertwined in many ways some of which we know and other ways which we are just beginning to discover.

Physiology is the scientific study of the functions and actions of an organism within its community and its ecosystem of which it is a part. And, of course, pathology is the study of the interferences to an organism's good health. Therefore, we urge every person to be responsible for knowing and understanding those inimical forces that are deleterious to individual and community health and wellness.

The principle function of physiology is the complex integration of the systems within the human body. Two major systems that affect our daily experience and functioning are the nervous system and the endocrine system. They play major roles in the reception and transmission of signals that integrate the complex functioning necessary for life. As new evidence emerges, we learn that biophotons and other forms of electromagnetic radiation play a major role in our physiology and health. A system in balance, in harmony with other systems is in homeostasis. This is an indicator of one's state of health.

Homeostasis is the maintenance of a stable internal environment, essential for life.[1] This means that we need to be internally balanced. There are many factors affecting homeostasis including oxygen and carbon dioxide concentrations, pH which is a measure of acidity or alkalinity in the body, salt and electrolyte concentrations, blood glucose concentrations, nutrient and waste product concentrations, intracellular and extracellular volume and pressure, body temperature, fluids, gradients and chemical environments in and around cell bodies. Basically, our greater than one hundred trillion cells are a social network aggregated into multiple communities, i.e., organs. These organs consist of types of cells with specialized functions. For example, red blood cells, approximately 25 trillion of them in each adult human body, specialize in oxygen transportation.[1] This organ works with the community of lung cells which make up the lung and specialize in diffusion of gases (oxygen in and carbon dioxide out). Our alveoli or functional units in the lungs operate opposite of the plant world (carbon dioxide in and oxygen out). In a broader homeostasis, we exist in a symbiosis with the plant world in this regard. Suffice it to say that homeostasis consists of multiple dynamic equilibrium scenarios in our bodies and with our environment and adjustment and regulation to these equilibria by the internal body systems and external environmental systems is necessary for good health.

There are three essential components to the maintenance of homeostasis. These are: a) sensory reception, or receiving information about the internal environment; b) integration of this sensory information, and c) the response to the original sensory stimuli. For example, you walk outside in the winter, the air is cold, and your skin feels the cold via sensory receptors in the skin. The brain processes this information and then selects a response; it decides to shiver to generate warmth. This instruction is then given to the muscle cells and the teeth begin chattering. The brain then sends messages of solution to the problem and directs the person-body to go indoors for additional clothing. The sensory receptors detect various stimuli which indicate fluctuations in the internal environment. These stimuli then are registered in the brain to formulate a response issued through effectors or muscles and glands. Endocrine glands, for example, which secrete hormones, have an effect aimed at countering the fluctuation and restoring the balance.

**Hydration: We are what we drink!**

Never mind the saying you are what you eat. More importantly, you are what you drink! Approximately fifty to seventy percent of ones total body weight is comprised of water. Fat tissue has lower water content relative to other body tissues,[2]—with more fat tissue, the less hydrated one becomes. So, for example, women tend to have a lower percent of their body weight as water because, relative to men, they have a higher percentage of fat than men, whereas obese individuals approach the extreme low end of the range.

So, approximately, sixty percent of one's total body weight is comprised of water. This total body water is divided into two main parts. About forty percent is intracellular and about twenty percent is extracellular. Of our extracellular water about seventy-five percent is predominantly surrounding and bathing our cells in what is called the interstitial space, with the remaining roughly twenty-five percent being in the blood plasma.[2] Amniotic fluid as well as intracellular fluid, interestingly, has salinity similar to ancient seawater, a harkening back to our primordial and primeval origins!

## Nutrition: Our bedrock!

Now to the proverbial you are what you eat. What comes from the air, soil, water and sunlight becomes you. You are a complex biological ecosystem built with and requiring constant replenishment of proteins and amino acids, carbohydrates, fats and fatty acids, vitamins, minerals, a diverse cornucopia of phytochemicals, and even photons, i.e., sunlight!

If the soil, air and water from which your food comes is devoid of these nutritional requirements your body will become deficient—it's that simple. The mounting scientific evidence agrees with common sense with regard to organic versus conventional food production. Organic food production, free of several toxins put on conventional crops, has been scientifically and conclusively demonstrated to lessen the chances of our getting a variety of unnecessary afflictions that we are predisposed to. The dangers of pesticides and herbicides among other toxins in our food supply seriously threaten our health status and contribute to the astronomical costs of disease care. Seriously, who wants petrochemicals and a multitude of other toxins in their food, in their food-chain, and in their neighborhood? These things ravage our health and the well-being of our ecosystems! While this chapter is not intended to provide and exhaustive overview of toxins we are exposed to on a daily basis, it becomes important to recognize the urgency of the situation. The following serves as testament to the gravity of what we face.

In a 2004 study by the Environmental Working Group, in collaboration with Commonweal, two major laboratories documented an average of 200 industrial toxicants in umbilical cord blood from 10 babies who were born August-September of 2004 in U.S. hospitals. Their tests demonstrate the presence of 287 chemicals in the cohort. Of these 287 chemicals detected, 180 cause cancer, 217 are neurotoxic, and 208 cause birth defects and abnormal development. The combined effects of these toxins have not been studied.[3]

Another telling study with regard to our ongoing environmental debacle is the Experimental Man Project, an in-depth scientific study into the presence of toxins and their effect upon the genes and physiology of one man who has elected to undergo the extensive testing. This far, out of 320 toxins tested for, he has tested positive for 165.[4] These efforts, in part are giving rise to a new science coined human envirogenomics or the fusing of environmental toxicology and genetics — two fields that until recently did not interact a whole lot with one another. From

these efforts science is once again showing a strong correlate to common sense —
toxins are detrimental to our health.

Mercury, a well-know toxic heavy metal, though banned from thermometers and
the environment, since it is extremely toxic even in minute quantities, continues
to be put in peoples' mouths in the form of dental amalgams. Fluoride added to
drinking water is another toxin! Another good example, is Cadmium (Cd), an
extremely toxic heavy metal used in a multitude of consumer goods including
batteries, paints, even jewelry. Heavy metals and various toxins exert their toxic
effects by interrupting normal physiology. For example, toxins displace of
essential minerals which then renders an altered physiology in the organism.
They also interfere with normal physiology by up regulating or down regulating
certain endocrine, or hormonal actions — dubbed endocrine disruptors. Heavy
metals and various plastics are notorious for endocrine disruption. Cd is
illustrative of this as it has been shown to mimic estrogens in breast cancer cell
lines and it has been shown to contribute to hormonal, in particular,
estrogen/progesterone imbalance.[5,6,7,8,9] There are a number of prominent
laboratories currently working on the issue of Cd induced disruption of
endocrine function, so much more data in this regard should be emerging. Also,
it should be mentioned that the indirect effects of Cd antagonism has been well
studied with regard to prostate and testicular cancer.

The question becomes, "well then what do we do?" We do not exist in a toxic
free world at present, however, on a planetary level we need to move more
toward this scenario with every available effort — truly we all need to come
together as a global people in this regard. In the meanwhile, on a personal level,
we must avoid as many toxins as possible and even undergo periodic cleansing
tailored to alleviate our toxic burdens and the sequestration of these toxins. And,
in addition to this, we must become educated about and engage in cleansing of
the internal body which has been commonplace in traditional societies for
millenia!

More than 80% of the world's populations' primary healthcare comes from
traditional healers![10] Taken together with the fact that approximately one in
every four modern day medical drugs stems from traditional healing
knowledge,[10,11] it becomes evident that indigenous technology works quite well.
These long-lived, healthful elders' philosophy and lifestyle practices, dietary and
nutritional practices, hold much wisdom. And, they reflect much of what we
know scientifically. Indeed, our leading causes of morbidity and mortality need
not exist because they are preventable by dietary and lifestyle modifications.

Serious ailments and their disease burdens could be reduced drastically including 70% of colon cancer, cerebral vascular accidents, coronary artery disease, and myocardial infarction (heart attack), and, 90% of diabetes type two.[12] And as traditional healers suggest, these lifestyle modifications include dietary practices of plant-based diets that are high in fiber and phytonutrients, low intakes of saturated and transfats, and low glycemic loads. Additional modifications include physical activity, brisk walking for greater than 30 min/day, nonsmoking, and a body mass index of less than 25 kg/meters-sq.

A convergence of independent research results also suggests nutrition can both reduce the risk for declining cognition and Alzheimer's disease as well as slow the progression of these debilitating ailments. Nancy Emerson Lombardo explains the scientific basis supplanting memory preservation nutrition, which is a comprehensive dietary program that applies these research results with older adults. Because of the nature of the nutritional program it also helps prevent and reverse diabetes and vascular diseases, which likely elevate the risk and accelerate the progression of Alzheimer's.[13]

Another example of traditional wisdom can be illustrated by the current explosion in interest in Vitamin D and health. Vitamin D, which is naturally present in very few foods, added to others in fortification processes, and available as a dietary supplement, is also produced endogenously as ultraviolet sunlight strikes our skin. The most physiologically active form is perhaps that which is derived from photosynthesis in our skin. There is a growing consensus that there are widespread and overlooked deficiencies among the general population. And, as we accelerate our scientific understanding of Vitamin D it becomes clear that its role in our maintenance of health is complex and multi-factorial. For example, we now know that in addition to the classic bone strength and health benefits, i.e., prevention of osteoporosis along with adequate calcium attributed to adequate Vitamin D, it has also been linked to possible prevention of various cancers,[14] diabetes type I,[15] and type II,[16] hypertension,[17] chronic pain,[18] multiple sclerosis,[19] and it modulates neuromuscular and immune function, reduction of inflammation, and the very cell cycle.[20,21,22,23]

Our traditional elders demonstrate that we need to spend more time outside. However, they also point out the importance of moderation. A meaningful note since the exposure of sunlight required for adequate Vitamin D synthesis is much less than the exposure that would bring on sunburn.[24,25]

Our longest-lived people are predominantly vegetarian or eat diets high in plant products and whole foods and low in animal products. They consume a diversity of freshly picked herbs, vegetables and fruits. The majority of their caloric intake is from fresh, raw vegetables. Sprouted items are common in their diets. They can easily identify herbs, vegetables and fruits with rejuvenating, healing qualities and they consume them regularly. They seldom eat refrigerated items, or foods laden with refined white flour, refined white sugar, preservatives, hydrogenated oils or processed foods of any kind. Their foodstuff is organic in the truest sense of the word, grown in areas high in ecological integrity, with nutrient rich soil and virtually devoid of chemical fertilizers, pesticides or herbicides. Every day they eat at the same time, regularly and in small proportions. By Western standards, their daily caloric intake would be considered sparse. However, their calorie-sparse foods are nutrient rich given their predominant fresh, raw, whole foods nature.

They do not involve themselves in lengthy, serious conversation while eating. Eating slowly and with intention is a part of their routine. For instance, one Indian said "each time you put food in the mouth we need to chew it thirty two times, once for each tooth." They consume large quantities of pure, fresh water, most often from local springs or pristine flowing water right from the earth. Their beverages are not commonly chilled, and are consumed often as teas, or in India, warm water with cumin seeds. They do not drink while they eat, only rarely and if then sparingly. They maintain optimal hydration throughout the day. Several types of herbs and spices are a regular part of their diet. Even if they need to travel to other places, they insist on eating at their regular times. They make it a point not to sleep or lie down at least two hours after they eat. Fasting is an integral part of their dietary patterns. Their practices vary mainly from one day per week to two weeks per year. And, if they imbibe in alcoholic beverages they do so with moderation. Fermented and cultured beverages are common.

We need to follow their example. With regular cleansing practices for detoxification one can achieve a healthy, energized physiology. The following are currently the most effective detoxification modalities: colonic irrigation, chlorella and algae, various herbals, saunas, especially infra-red, lymphatic drainage, acupuncture, chelation, and zeolites.[26]

It is found in ancient Sanskritic texts, preached in the practices of Hinduism, Buddhism, Taoism and a number of other traditional practices the world over: We must conceive of our bodies and treat our bodies as a temple.

Our bodies derive from a sacred act of creation. Our bodies must be sacrosanct, protected from the pollution and toxins now encroaching upon everyday life and which degrade the body and detract from one's quality of life and innate abilities at health. We must be aware of those agents that interfere with the potentialities we all possess. Our knowledge of what hurts us and what helps us will provide ourselves and our communities with a wealth that cannot be measured in dollars.

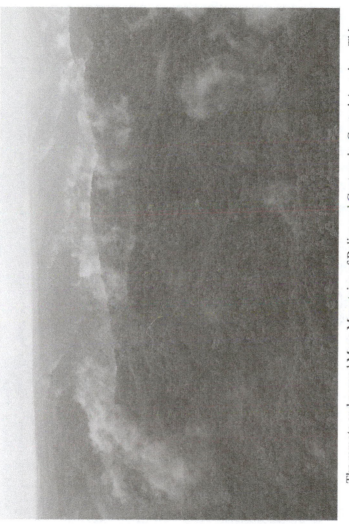

The remote and rugged Maya Mountains of Belize and Guatemala, Central America. This area is a biodiversity hotspot. Most of the Maya Mountains in Belize have been designated a protected area. These mountains are home to the Traditional Q'eqchi' Maya Healers and Itzama.

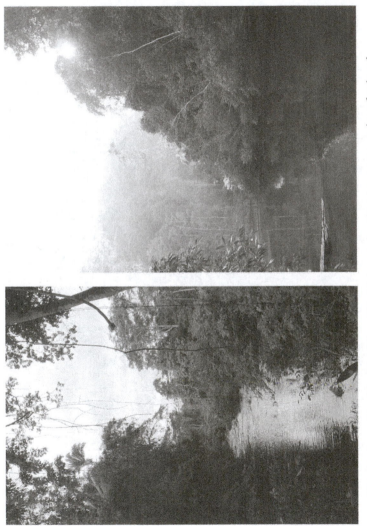

The riparian networks of the Maya Mountains are host to numerous species of cultural and medicinal import.

Plant collections are conducted by the Q'eqchi' Maya healers in the riparian networks of the Maya Mountains and thousands of plants representing over 200 species have been successfully transplanted to their garden at Itzama.

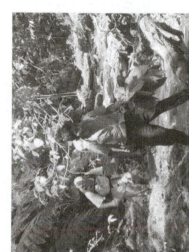

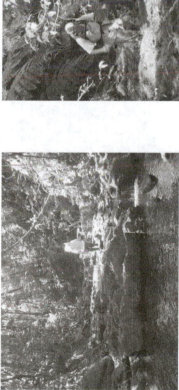

Innovation in irrigation techniques are essential for the growth of certain species. The garden is outside of the pristine primary rainforest of the Maya Mountains and therefore there are requirements such as moisture, shade, and companion plants which need to be accommodated at the garden. Note the planting of certain species on or around the tree-fall and tree-stumps to control for these moisture and humus content variables to promote healthful plant growth.

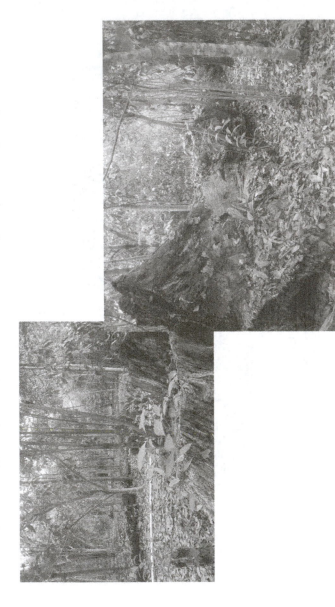

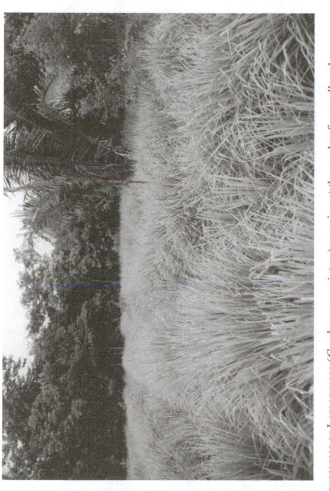

Fevergrass or Lemongrass (*Cymbopogon ciatrus*) growing at the garden for small scale commercialization. This is one of the popular medicinal plants in Belize, and indeed the world, and is used for fevers, cold and flu.

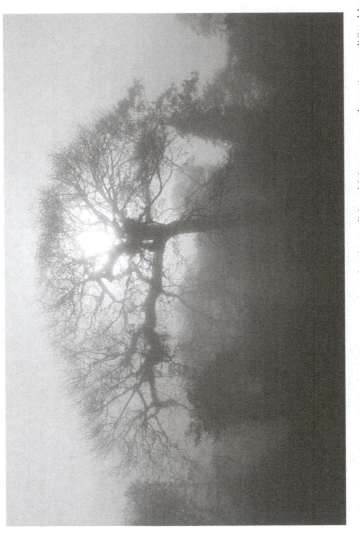

The *Yaxche* "Tree of Life" (*Ceiba pentandra*), for the traditional Maya means the *axis mundi* "stable world center" which connects the terrestrial and spirit worlds.

Envisioning Itzama workshop where the healers and partners planned the initiation and development of cultural healing center and gardens. Resultant from the workshop was an action plan on the development of Itzama as well as first steps at integrating traditional healing with national healthcare, the careful planning involving the community from the outset has been instrumental in the success of Itzama.

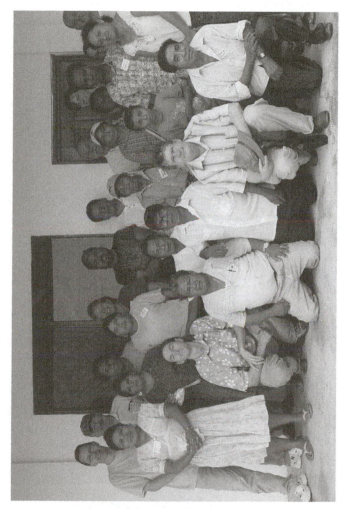

Authors discussing the Itzama Model with Muthuvan and Uraly elders and healers of the Western Ghats, Kerala, India, another biodiversity hotspot. The Itzama Model is being implemented there now in a novel indigenous peoples technology exchange program facilitated through the Center for Healing Across Cultures.

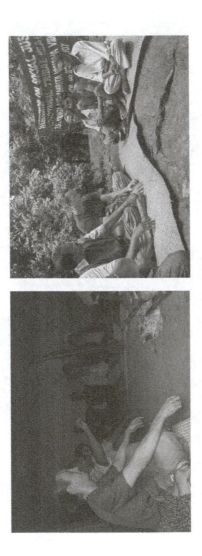

We must act quickly the world over in revival of our healing traditions and our connection to the natural world in health. Just as there is action and need in the biodiversity hotspots of the Maya Mountains, Belize, and Western Ghats, India, there is action and need in your back yard. Whoever you are, wherever you are, you can get started. For example, Appalachian herbalists in Appalachian Mountains of eastern U.S. working to repatriate Ginseng (*Panex quinquefolius*), a local medicinal plant almost extirpated due to unsustainable harvesting for commercial demands. The U.S. has been exporting Ginseng internationally since the 1700's. If a percentage of these profits made it back to the mountains, there would be much more protected for future generations.

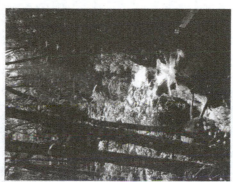

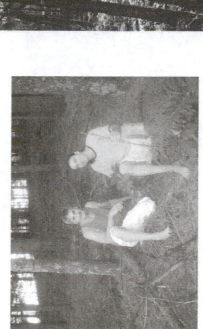

Support your local, organic, sustainable growers and herbalists markets whether in India, Andean or Amazonian Peru, or right at home. Food is our medicine!

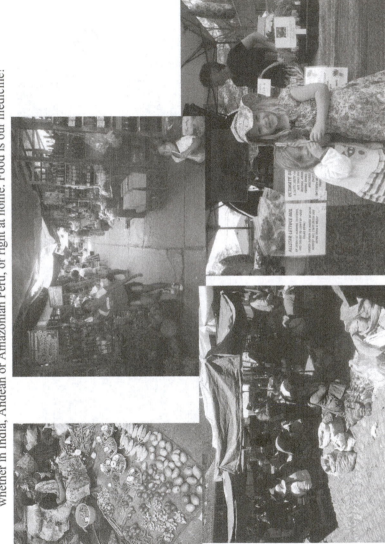

# Chapter 4
# Mind: It Isn't Just in Your Head

*"It is believed by most that time passes; in actual fact, it stays where it is."*

**Dogen**

*"The eyes only see what the mind is prepared to comprehend."*

**Henri Bergson**

*"The influence of the senses have in men overpowered the thought to the degree that the walls of time and space have come to look solid, real and insurmountable... Yet time and space are but inverse measures of the power of the mind. Man is capable of abolishing them both."*

**Ralph Waldo Emerson**

People's common conceptions of the mind most often locate it in the brain/head, with connections to the heart. They think of it as a consciousness that reasons, thinks, feels, wills, perceives, experiences based on input and emotion, and judges internal and external states of being. It includes intellect or understanding and appreciating, opinion, viewpoints, sentiment, inclination, intention, and desire. It includes attention and intention, and conceptualizations of spirituality would also be a valid inclusion.

**Brain and Mind**

Some random points about brain and mind:

- The brain weighs three pounds and consists of 60% fat.[1]

- Every heartbeat provides 25% of your blood and oxygen to the brain.[1]

- The brain consists of 1.1 trillion cells, including 100 billion neurons.[2]

- A typical neuron fires 5-50 times per second and within a few seconds quadrillions of signals will travel throughout the brain.[2] Each of these signals are a quantum of information and the totality of these quanta or information is what we may call mind.

- The number of combinations of 100 billion neurons firing or not firing is 10 to the millionth power, or 10 followed by a million zeros.[2] This is the number of possible states of the brain and/or mind. The number of atoms in the universe is estimated to be 10 to the 80th power.[2]

- The brain is a stimulus and response system to the organism of the body. The stimulus and response system reaches out into the world of nature and culture and the electromagnetic and other fields of our cosmic surroundings.

- The brain is perhaps the primary, but not the only generator and shaper of the mind.

- There are greater than 100 trillion living cells in the human body each of which generates an electrochemical field, all of which create a superconductive electrochemical field that transmits and receives energy and communicative intelligence throughout and beyond the body.

- The brain/mind has the ability to generate molecules of emotion.

- The separate concepts "mind" and "body" is a false dichotomy.

- There exists a distribution of cellular intelligence throughout the human body. An example of cellular memory: In her book, *Change of Heart*, the author, Claire Sylvia, received a heart from a man killed in a motorcycle accident. Shortly after her transplant she took a great liking for motorcycles and beer![3]

- There are four general levels of mind: the unconscious, subconscious, conscious, and superconscious mind.

- We have evolved the ability to download an unimaginable number of behaviors, beliefs, emotional states, and predispositions into our memory at these aforementioned four levels of the mind.

- The conscious mind processes 40 environmental stimuli per second.

- The subconscious mind processes 20,000,000 environmental stimuli per second which is 500,000 times greater than the conscious mind.

- Certain states of heightened consciousness enable us to experience information from the unconscious, which has a more expansive perspective of reality since it is not filtered by the brain.[4]

- The superconscious is spirit energy, the quantum physics of mentation and being.

- As evidenced by psychic phenomena such as telepathy, precognition, and clairvoyance, as well accessing information via dreams and out of body experiences provides evidence that mentation and consciousness exists outside of the brain/body.[4]

**Barriers to Consciousness: The Ego-Mechanisms of Defense**

Psychoanalysis has also provided us with information on another dimension of the mind, mechanisms that shield the conscious mind from emotional pain, distress and perhaps even constructs of reality in instances that may not confer survival advantage to humans. These are termed the ego-mechanisms of defense. They are processes that we can postulate are lawful principles of the mind/body, perhaps conveying survival advantage or stability to the organism which then promotes survival advantage.

The process generally starts with deprivation or other stimuli which cause the experience of frustration or helplessness which inevitably leads to a level of hostility which results in a disposition to aggression at which point the individual makes a conscious or unconscious decision on how to express the experience. These psychological processes limit the level of consciousness an individual may actualize, and although protecting the individual from emotional pain, create disruptions in the harmony and equanimity of the mind. Within the framework of the theory of psychoanalysis the mechanism of repression is the primary process that mobilizes the other ego-defense mechanisms. Repression is the shunting of an experience into the realm of the unconscious. Once the impulse pattern of the experience is rendered unconscious other ego-defense mechanisms can come into play.

Denial is a common ego-defense mechanism that may come into play when one experiences a stressful, objectionable, distasteful, or an anxiety-producing situation. A common example is when a husband hears his wife's complaints or angry expressions of a situation the husband may be involved in and the husband dismisses her discomfort as a "female thing" rather than seriously listening to her complaint and empathically understanding the rift in their relationship. Another example, is one of overly skeptical professional opinions "its not what I learned therefore its not correct."

Displacement is the ego-defense mechanism whereby an act of aggression is directed against a target that was not the source of one's frustration. An example is a man who is publically humiliated by his boss but cannot act on his boss's abuse; goes home where wife complains he didn't take out the garbage and he inappropriately releases his rage upon her; and she then inappropriately screams at her child who just came into the house without taking off his shoes. The individuals in this situation may not have been aware of the level of rage that had built up and so acted impulsively, serving their own ego needs without concern for the target of their rage, which, of course, disrupts the harmony and love of the relationship and community—local and global.

Another ego-defense mechanism that is generated by deprivation leading to frustration and hostility is involution. Involution is, for our purposes here, anger turned inward. In this state the person may not be aware of the process operating. If there is no feasible way to express the frustration and anger, the angry mind will turn it inward and process it there. In this case turning anger inward may be directed in toward the self or turning the anger against one's own group or perceived group or antithetic group. Involution occurs, for example, in shame of one's ethnic identity, lack of awareness or connection to ones cultural identity or heritage, and preconceived notions or prejudice to name a few. And, oftentimes involution manifests in rage such as violence, especially when the source of the deprivation or frustration lies outside the group. This anger turned inward has two routes of mental expression as well: the emotional pathway is recognized as anxiety and depression while the psychosomatic route manifests in physical ailments commonly connected to stress responses. These physical manifestations normally include symptoms such as headaches or migraines, heart palpitations, stomach or esophageal hyperacidity—leading to ulcers, gastroenteritis, colitis, severe depression, severe anxiety, heart disease, and cancer. It can also include prolonged periods of sadness, insomnia, fatigue, feeling "slowed down", decreased sexual vitality, periods of sadness interspersed with hyperinflated emotional feelings (or mania), self-destructive acts, or suicidal ideation. There is a tendency for females to experience depression and males to manifest psychosomatic symptoms, although this difference can change with the change in cultural conditions, as in the masculinization of women. Involution or "bottled up anger" can fester in the body/mind and virtually "eat one up".

The reaction-formation defends against a repressed unacceptable impulse and converts it into its opposite. An example: a young man feels, often unconsciously, he hasn't lived up to the masculine ideals of his culture and feels effeminate. The emotional reaction is fear of this taboo impulse. To react against this impulse he will over-react and play the machismo role expressing hyper-masculinity.

Fixation is a response, often experienced in one's developing years, that prevents the individual further emotional growth. Failure of continued growth and development may occur as a result of a severely traumatic experience or pattern of traumatic experiences, such as harsh punishment, severe physical injury, early childhood sexual or other abuse, extremely painful initiation ceremonies such as unanaesthetized circumcision or clitoridectomy and infibulation practiced in certain indigenous cultures of Africa and the Middle East, or even circumcision practiced in Western cultures.

Associated with the intrapersonal repression and fixation is the social aspect that we identify as identity foreclosure where an individual, still in the stage of development and maturation, has no proper role models to identify with and continue in the maturation process; where an individual is entirely dependent on their peer group for identification and sustenance for role-modeling. Gang membership is one such example, pathological cult groups, another. What is critical to recognize is that it is the emotional level of development of that person's identity that will be foreclosed. It is sometimes heard that men about to marry are dragged out of their adolescence kicking and screaming into the adulthood of responsibility and commitment!

It is important to note here that the aforementioned ego-defense mechanisms can be nullified, in part, along with varied states of longing, loneliness and despair through cultural practices replete with respect and reverence of our elders, our heritage, and nature. In essence these are grounding for our children and provide calming sustenance and "roots." This grounding, in turn, enables opening of the mind and a sort of clearing of the "clutter" toward the cultivation of consciousness.

Opening the mind depends on one having awareness of and control over those events that trigger the ego-defense mechanisms and that create distortions of perception, convolutions of cognition, and anger-driven behavior in relationships. Opening the mind creates a broader horizon of consciousness, a deeper awareness, and an empathic sensitivity to others and the environment.

And, very importantly, an opened mind can channel potentially destructive impulses into creative efforts that benefit the self, the community, and the environment within which one lives. How we do this is discussed in the next chapter.

## The Structural Levels of the Mind

We like to think of the mind in terms of several levels of functioning—here we enumerate five: conscious, subconscious, unconscious, deep mind of cellular intelligence, and beyond these levels which is the super-mind or super-consciousness.

The conscious mind needs little elaboration. It is our momentary awareness of what we are perceiving, thinking, feeling and doing.

The subconscious mind is that realm that is easily retrievable into the conscious mind with the proper cues, such as "Did you smell something burning?" or "I wonder how your dog is right now?" or when asked "What did you eat for breakfast yesterday?". The unconscious mind stores material both cognitive and emotional, not easily retrievable unless in heightened consciousness. It might be memory traces from birth or infancy, or painful experiences that one wishes not to remember, or the myriad of situations, events, and relationships that are too numerous to easily remember or remember at all.

We consider "deep mind" as the totality of life-energy structures, processes, and functions that we are not aware of but contribute to our life-experience at any moment in time. Structures within a living cell communicate with each other and regulate life-giving functions; configurations of cells are integrated and communicate within organs to maintain organic functioning, and the super-regulatory organ, the brain, communicates with the organismic structures of the body; all inform us that this communication, this intraorganismic integration and response, this maintenance of intraorganismic balance or homeostasis, is manifest as intelligence, cellular intelligence. For example, when we get a cut in the skin, the surrounding cells get the message, essentially instantaneously and know what to do to begin the process of inflammation and then some to heal the wound. That is a mode of adaptation resulting from the signals, the messages that are conveyed by the injured cells.

We do not want to stop here in articulating our conception of mind thus we introduce biophotonic energy and its corresponding biophotonic energy of the mind. Biophotons are the smallest physical units of light. They are electromagnetic radiation in the visible spectrum. They are absorbed by, emitted by, stored by and utilized by all the biological organisms on this planet. The food we eat, especially raw foods, most importantly, vegetables, transport these transporters of energy, viz., biophotons, into our cells. These biophotons contain important information that controls the vital processes that order and regulate cellular functioning, keep us alive, energized, promoting vitality and wellbeing.

Every living organism emits biophotons defined as low-level luminescence, normally with wavelengths of 200 and 800 nanometers. It is believed, that the higher the luminescence emission the greater its vitality and the greater the potential for the transfer of that energy to the organism consuming it.

The biophotonic emissions of the body come from the vibrations of our DNA. The DNA within each of our cells vibrates at a frequency of several billion hertz. This vibration is created through the coil-like contractions of the DNA, occurring several billion times per second. With these contractions it emits biophotons, as does all matter. It is believed that all the biophotons emitted from an organism communicate with each other in a highly structured light field surrounding the body—this field provides near instantaneous communication. This light field regulates the activity of the metabolic enzymes. This phenomenon most certainly borders on the mystical: each cell's DNA vibrates at several billion hertz, several billion times per second, multiplied by greater than one hundred trillion living cells with the human body. It manifests an intelligence the likes of which we have yet to fully understand and appreciate.

The super-conscious mind is a concept not well understood nor accepted by a great proportion of scientists. Astrophysicists speak of the "grid" of the universe; lines of energy that influence astronomical bodies and living creatures. The artist Alex Grey paints these lines of energy in his works of human beings. It is a notion that provides for us a vehicle for the cognitive and emotional connection of us all.

**Instinctual predisposition to alter the mind's consciousness: Ritual and Therapeutic Methodologies and Botanical Technologies**

We maintain that there is a natural predisposition to alter one's state of consciousness and condition of one's mind. We can conceive changing states of mind on a continuum from very mundane and ordinary to exciting to extremes of ecstasy and orgasmic love to terror, shock, and dissociation. Deep sleep and dreaming are states of mind. Commensality with good friends and a fine meal creates a certain state of mind. Being moved by a powerful drama or meeting someone you missed and hadn't seen in some time are other states of mind. Sunrise, sunset, walk in the woods all induce altered states of mind and cultivation of consciousness. Falling in love or experiencing betrayal are powerful states of mind. An encounter with a threat, physical or psychological, generates a strong endocrine/physiologic response and the attending emotional state of mind.

Therefore, altered states of consciousness can be accidental and involuntary, as with surprise, or strong connections with people or places, or even finding a great *entre* on a menu you didn't expect. Or, altered states can be voluntary where one prepares oneself for an altered experience. This can be with the aid of ritual involving psychotropic substances used through millennia of the human experience. Humanity has always facilitated expanded/altered states of consciousness through imbibing in plants or fungi with psychotropic properties. Or, it can be with a voluntary preparation engendered by directed thought, fasting, sensory quiescence, chanting, song, drumming or other rhythmic oscillation of sound, dance, postures, controlled breathing, isolation, meditation, or any combination of these and then some! It appears that the practice of a variety of meditation modalities has far-reaching therapeutic effects on a person and the group.

**The Yoga Mind**

In the yoga sutras of Patanjali it is stated that the yoga mind is the cessation of the busyness and fluctuations and free-flying imagery of the normal mind. It is, essentially, the cessation of the continuous flow of thought, which interjects fluctuations in consciousness, to provide for a state of being closer to pure uninterrupted consciousness. The yoga teacher, Karen Allgire, contrasts *citta-vrttis*, the incessant mental activity, with *narodha*, restraint, control, and stilling of the mind's activities, which can then lead us into a deep, inner peace.[5] With meditative practice, this experienced moment of inner peace will gradually infuse the rest of one's life and allow one to live their life in a clearer, more balanced way, not influenced or polluted by toxic thoughts and feelings or prejudicial notions that distort the existential reality. As Karen Allgire points out in Patanjali's sutras, the five states of mind, the *citta-vrttis*, that disturb our perception and inhibit deep inner peace are: *viparyaya* or the illusion of misperception; *vikalpa* or delusion, fantasy, or thoughts based on illusion that do not have their basis in reality; *nidra*, or deep dreamless sleep that does not correspond to existential reality; *smrtih*, or memory, which is a source of knowledge and discrimination, but may also keep one in a state of nostalgia or regret, which is not a state of existential reality, or in a state of mistaken or distorted past realities. The state of *pramana* is that of correct perception and accurate understanding of reality. This state of consciousness allows us to encounter a person, place, object, statement, scent, or action without preconception, stereotypy, prejudice, association with a past event, or wrongful teaching.

A demonstration of *pramana* and its antithetical state can be illustrated by the following: Once upon a time, Dr. Reminick (one of the authors) owned an eighteen-foot, 140 pound Burmese python. It was quite docile and his children played with it for years, under the supervision of their father. Mr. Burmese Python made many trips to daycare centers, public schools, and a few college classes. He would be carried in a large red leather trunk, put on the table with a few moments of introduction and commentary. The presenter's children, at one point aged 8 and 10 were most-always present. When the trunk was opened Mr. Burmese Python would raise his head, extend himself, something like a cobra, and proceed to cascade out of the trunk on to the table and flow onto the floor. It was always a rather spectacular sight. The author's two boys would then pet it, sit on it, and play. Then the other kids would join in. The teachers, on the other hand would back off with their backs pressed to the wall (wondering why they invited the author in the first place) in shock. Then the point was made: The children had no preconception, no learned fear, no pre-judging of the situation. They saw there was no danger and were free to enjoy this creature of nature. The teachers, on the other hand, had learned about snakes and were conditioned by their preconceptions and their prejudgments, their prejudice, and were therefore, fearful. The point was made, how preconceiving something, prejudging something, without the confirmation of existential experience, can produce unnecessary fear and wrongful behavior in people ignorant of the reality they encounter. The state of *narodha* could have allowed them to enjoy, learn, and appreciate the phenomenon before them.

Yoga *asanas* or postures, yoga breathing, and the yoga state of mind all bring the gift of mindfulness and presence to the practitioner. It brings deep relaxation to the person allowing us to be quiet yet aware, calm yet attentive, slowed down to perceive deeply into one's core and then outward to the cosmos; to gain insight into who one really is, it allows us to be fully in the moment and to appreciate the life within our present and without our experience or its surrounding clutter.

## Meditation Medicine

As Western medical practitioners begin to understand the mind's role in health and disease, there has been more interest in the use of meditation in medicine and psychotherapy. In fact, the field of psychoneuroimmunology has found that the immune system is not static in its performance. Research in this field has shown that it is greatly influenced by our neurology, and that we are now discovering the relationship between thoughts, emotions and health. We are also learning of the positive effects of meditation in healing a variety of afflictions caused by stress.[6]

Meditative practices are increasingly offered in medical clinics and hospitals as a tool for improving health and quality of life, as is the case with Kabat-Zinn's "Stress Reduction and Relaxation Center" in Massachusetts. Meditation has been used as the primary therapy for treating certain diseases; as an additional therapy in a comprehensive treatment plan; and as a means of improving the quality of life of people with debilitating or chronic pain, those with terminal illnesses, such as cancer, or those suffering from AIDS.[7]

In Kabat-Zinn's center, patients reported that during meditation, chronic pain was 40-50% less severe. This is a phenomenon more fully discussed by Austin[7] where he talks of the ways in which the body deals with pain. He reviews a study where a Yogi lied on a bed of nails, while meditating. The investigator attempted this, and could not tolerate the discomfort. When they both used naloxone to counter any opioid effects (many pain relievers act at opioid receptors in the brain, where morphine exerts its action), their pain toleration levels did not change. This showed that there is some non-opioid effect that occurs during meditation. While it has not been fully explained or explored as to where in the mind this occurs, or how or why, it is sufficient to infer that meditation helps relieve or cancel the pain response. Another research example is a study by Barnes.[8] Forty-five African American adolescents that were having behavior issues in school were divided into 2 groups. In the experimental group they practiced 15-minute sessions of Transcendental Meditation at home and at school. The control group had that time filled with the basic "health class" material. The students' number of rule infractions, absentee periods, suspension days due to behavioral issues, all significantly decreased in the experimental group compared to an increase in the control group. Research in schools has also found that meditation may be helpful for teachers.[9] Winzelberg was concerned about the high burnout rates and stress levels found in teachers. Their stress symptoms included emotional and behavioral pathology and gastronomic distress. He constructed an experiment to see if meditation would be an effective way to ease this problem. The researchers instructed teachers in the techniques of relaxation response and guided them through the meditation process involving mantras, slowing down one's actions, and one-pointed attention. It was found that the teachers in the experimental group were able to effectively reduce their stress symptoms. An illustrative case study is demonstrated by David Shannahoff-Khalsa[10] involving a 20-year-old college woman. She began working with David during her university's spring break of 2001, in hopes of reducing her social anxiety, academic stress, body dysmorphic disorder (BDD), obsessive-compulsive disorder (OCD), and depression. The patient said that she really felt she was struggling in life and yet after the first session her BDD and OCD both disappeared for the duration of the day. Despite that astounding progress, after spring break, class resumed and she ceased her meditation and, consequently, relapsed into her former symptomatology. As her pathology progressed she would spend 2 hours each day in front of the mirror, convinced the right side of her face was distorted. A psychiatrist prescribed Fluoxetine (a Selective Serotonin Reuptake Inhibitor or SSRI), but it only deepened the issues she was having by making her anxious and depressed. She developed new symptoms of smoking and self-mutilation. In some cases when she cut her arms, she needed several stitches because of the deep lacerations. Her parents also noticed that she was beginning to show symptoms of anorexia. She would eat only 1 meal per day and was rapidly losing weight. In 2002 she was hospitalized and then taken back to her therapist, David. After meeting with him again, she replaced her medication with yoga. As a result, like the previous meditation therapy, her condition immediately improved. She was able to quit smoking and stop the self-mutilation, and her appetite returned. With continued practice she has been able to maintain a greater state of peace and general strength that has continued up to the day of the article's publication. The above case demonstrates how emotionally-based symptoms can be alleviated.

In this second case, an immune-deficiency disease, dermatomyositis, was treated with meditation.[11] Dermatomyositis is a muscle disease that is characterized by a rash and muscle weakness, with the possibility of dysphagia (problems with swallowing). Eventually, people that suffer from this have a loss of strength, including difficulty getting up from a seated position, lifting objects, and climbing stairs. Treatment usually consists of prescribing a steroid drug, oftentimes accompanied by immunosuppressants and physical therapy to preserve muscle function. However in the case study conducted by Collins and Dunn, the only treatments used were meditation and visual imagery. During the course of observation progress with skin conditions were affected by stress, but strength was not. After meditation, the rash lessened and pain diminished. By the end of the 294-day observation period, she had healed her symptoms on her own. It is important to note that the mortality rate for dematomyositis is roughly 61% if left untreated, and the odds for "spontaneous recoveries" are rare. This shows that therapies that reinforce the mind-body connection are useful for treating this condition, and may be useful for treating others as well. Lastly, in Afari's twin study of chronic fatigue syndrome (CFS)[12] "twins with CFS were more likely to use homeopathy, mega-vitamins, herbal therapies, biofeedback, relaxation/meditation, guided imagery, massage therapy, energy healing, religious healing by others, and self-help groups than their non-CFS counterparts." This study also showed that the majority of the control and experimental research groups found these techniques to be helpful, with 81% for those suffering from CFS, and 71% for those without.

The authors, Drs. Pesek, Reminick and Nair, conducted a semester long study of university students contesting a control group to a Mindfulness Meditation intervention group via the Hamilton Anxiety Scale, a measure of anxiety. The intervention group was taught some Mindfulness Meditation techniques including belly breathing and clearing the mind. They were taught based on Jon Kabat-Zinn's [6] Seven Essential Attitudes as being a Foundation for Mindfulness, these are: Nonjudging, Patience, Beginner's Mind, Trust, Nonstriving, Acceptance, Letting Go. They were given instruction at the outset of the semester and they then practiced 5-10 minutes of Mindfulness Meditation several times per week throughout the semester (approximately 8 weeks) thereafter. The intervention group demonstrated a statistically significant 50% reduction in their Hamilton Anxiety Scale scores relative to that of the control group which was essentially unchanged.

**The Shamanic Mind and State of Consciousness**

Shamanic practitioners derive information while in deep trance. This information is generally about diagnosis, treatment of afflictions, divining future events, or finding solutions to the problems people bring to them. Although anthropologists often use the terms trance and ecstasy interchangeably, Tedlock[13] prefers to differentiate between the two. According to Barbara Tedlock trance is a "hyperlucid state of sensory overstimulation triggered by music, noises and odors". The experiences of trance states are often forgotten after one emerges into normalcy. In contrast, ecstasy is a state of sensory deprivation, withdrawing from the immediately perceivable world via fasting, total silence, meditation in complete darkness. Tedlock asserts that ecstatic experiences are not only remembered, they can be revisited over and over again. Examples of the latter include dreaming, tuning in to the body's vital energy or chi flows, or altered states produced by ingesting psychotropic substances or other activities. Powerful ways of bringing on trance states include drumming — repetitive, long-lasting, constant beats with concerted focus, and, chanting repeatedly with constancy brings many practitioners into the trance state. In Tedlock's experience of shamanic performances, her own and of other shamans, "participants may stamp their feet to one rhythm, clap their hands to a second rhythm, and sing syllables to yet a third".

Many anthropologists have seen how music that urges dancing profoundly alters the structure of one's consciousness, changing how one experiences both space and time. "Musically driven movements enable shamans and their clients to enter into spiritual worlds filled with culturally appropriate cosmic imagery". Participants will often dance to exhaustion, feeling exhilarated, ecstatic, renewed, joyful, and euphoric. Intense dancing leads to hyperventilation, increases the production of adrenaline, causes a sharp decrease in blood glucose stimulating the brain to mobilize the opiate-like endorphins and untold other effectors that surge through the body creating wonderful feelings of coursing energy rising up from the belly in waves creating an emotional expansiveness.

The many forms of constant, rhythmic percussion, such as with drums, rattles, or gongs, produce the phenomenon of entrainment. Entrainment occurs when the asynchronous patterns of brain waves come into harmonic resonance. Normally, in the waking state, one hemisphere of the brain dominates the other in an asynchronous pattern. Normally, the right hemisphere generates alpha waves, vibrating at seven to fourteen cycles per second. The left hemisphere generates beta waves vibrating at fourteen to twenty-one cycles per second. As neurophysiological research has shown, rhythmic sounds can alter brain wave patterns, produce entrainment, and induce the state of trance. Researchers of the brain call this process "sonic driving" which can produce visual patterns of color and movement and full-blown hallucination.

A common practice producing an altered/heightened state of consciousness is the use of entheogens, meaning "God generated within", plants, plant products or fungi that produce "mind expansion". There are hundreds of plants that shamans and healers, as well as others, use to induce altered state of consciousness, a change in mind. The more commonly known entheogens used for healing, shamanic ritual and other spiritual purposes, include cannabis, peyote, fly agaric, a mushroom used at least since the bronze age by peoples of

Siberia, as evidenced in their ancient rock art, North India, among the Greeks, Scandinavians, and Saami nomads of Lapland and many others; it is commonly found in the birch, fir, and pine forests of North Asia; and the birch, pine, and cedar forests of North America. Lewis Carroll may have had fly agaric in mind when he wrote "Alice in Wonderland" since Alice shrinks eating one side of the mushroom and stretches eating the other side. Similarly, in Walt Disney's "Snow White and the Seven Dwarfs they danced around fly agaric mushrooms.[14] We can also include psilocybin mushrooms, San Pedro cactus, and tobacco as commonly used entheogens among healers and shamans to alter one's state of consciousness. Lastly, we note the use of a plant called *qat* (Arabic) or *ch'at* (Amharic) the leaves of which are chewed by peoples of Islamic East Africa, including Sudan, Ethiopia, and Somalia, and many peoples of the Middle East. It is a mild alkaloid that allows one to remain awake all night, dampen the appetite, and provide boosts in energy reserves often used in ritual contexts. It bears a remarkable similarity to coffee and the ritual consumption of xanthine alkaloids (caffeine) its consumption brings, i.e., coffee with friends. It should also be noted, that one of the most powerful, if not the most powerful psychotropic substance known to occur in the plant/fungi world, is also endogenously produced in our brains. The substance, N,N-Dimethyltryptamine (DMT) is released in small amounts into our brain at various times including dreamtime.

Here, we will not include those hallucinogens that are used for recreational activities.

A more extreme altered state of consciousness requires the careful guidance of an experienced shaman, one type, is an *ayahuasquero*, who prepares the client, sometimes for several months before the ritual, for the ayahuasca experience. The phytochemicals in this Amazonian vine, mixed with other highly potent entheogens and companion plants, create some of the most powerful and colorful and dramatic experiences known to the human condition. It can transform a person; catapult them into exotic space; often finding freedom from the issues that held them back from insight into one's self, happiness, and potentiality. It is also a very powerful purgative and the participants become cleansed through bouts of diarrhea and vomiting.

A quote from an interview with an educated, middle-aged woman, yoga practitioner/teacher who traveled to Amazonia and engaged in the ritual of ayahuasca:

*"So we walked through the day, terrified; agreeing that this is good; and we're not being flippant about this; and came to sunset and entered this amazing sacred hut in the valley. And there were no windows, just a round candle-lit hut. And then this wizened old man walks in with his grandchild, about 8; his skin is leather; wrinkles and wrinkles and wrinkles; the beauty of this human being; his eyes! And he went around the room and looked each of us in the eyes; and his grandchild sat waiting for him. She carried the bucket of the brew. Alberto said, last night the brew was from the new part of the bark and not very strong. This is ancient and it will taste different, it will smell different, it will go down different. And you are required to drink a whole glass. I looked at John across the room. Looked here and there; Jim wasn't doing it…Alberto repeated, "If you consider this a drug experience, you will miss out. Especially you old druggies, you will miss out. So when the experience begins to get really intense, maybe in a half hour, and the ride begins, with the psychedelic experience; you will have to stay focused. Those of you with a yoga background you will fare well, because of your breathing. Do not let go of your breathing! I said, I'm golden, I got the tools. Let 'er go!*

*The shaman went first. Then Alberto took the drink. Then next was me. He blessed me, and by the time we got almost around to the person sitting on the other side of the room to me, I started feeling it. Tingling in my fingers and my toes, my eyesight started to be weird, blurry, and I said I guess its time to close my eyes. And I began to trip out. I was so nauseous I knew I was gonna puke on my own body! How disgusting was that! I remembered to b r e a t h e; and the vomit would get up to my throat and I would exhale and made it go down. And each time I breathed I would root myself. I was sitting in lotus; I can't sit comfortably in lotus more than 15 minutes, so I knew I wasn't gonna be in lotus for very long, but I didn't know how I was sitting because the ride, where I was sitting, was so intense that the lights and stream of lights…I couldn't hold on to anything. I was being dragged and nauseous; dragged from one light stream to another and I just kept breathing. I just kept saying to myself, breathe, breathe. Occasionally I heard Alberto's voice. The shaman walked around, rattling leaves, not even dry leaves; and rattled and chanted in front of us. And that kept me focused. It could have been the first hour, I dropped into another place. When the shaman stood in front of me, I heard him say — now he didn't speak any English — I heard him say, "State your intention!" Loud. He was in front of me. "My intention for healing is to heal every misperception in this lifetime and every other lifetime and having gotten that I want to go to the source of my beginning and once I've gotten that I want to be with God. And I said it over and over and over again. At that point I was so sick I said "I better open my eyes to see where the door is, because if I have to go out of here to throw up or have diarrhea I want to know where the door is! I gotta know where I am!" I opened my eyes and what I saw were these huge scorpions walking around the room. And I said, "Not safe out there!" Closed my eyes.*

*If I threw up it was going on my lap. I don't know what those things are, but I ain't goin'!" So I closed my eyes again and the scorpions went away. I started to travel into different realms and different life beings and different forms of life. At one point I was in, what looked like a rocket ship. The beings in the rocket ship, and I was one, big heads, bald heads and they didn't look human. I was – everything was fast! Just fast! Like I was soaring through realms of existence; going through and through and through; streaks and streams of light; there was – the light was me; I was light energy. I went in to the earth, into rock formations; I was experiencing on a tactual, sensation level; other realms of existence; a blade of grass, I could taste it – on a cellular level! And I was – at that point I was going so fast and I remember, shoo! I wish I could control this! Slow down! But I couldn't. And that went on – I don't know how long that went on. It could've been a long time; it could've been minutes. I was in a timeless realm! And then after that bouncing through all of these realms, occasionally I would hear the shaman, the rattle, and I would hear him say, "State your intention!"*

*Even in this stream I could state my intention; and I could breathe, so I knew I was in control of the situation. ... I felt safe; I was scared, but I felt safe. And all of a sudden things started to slow down enough for me to say, "Huh, I could ride this wave! Ok! This is ok. I must be in a different phase now. And in front of me was this enormous man, like from the Arabian Nights; with these flowing skirts wrapped around him and a big turban. He was a beautiful, beautiful black man. And in his hand he was carrying a book. And it was so heavy – and he's a huge being, but it weighs a lot. And the book opens up in front of me. And you know in those old movies the pages flow and they are going that fast; and I know that every page is a lifetime and every single page is a misperception of that lifetime! And I am in ecstasy, because it is I who am about to receive everything I came for! I'm going to heal every misperception from every lifetime as a human personality. And it's awesome, it's awesome. And I don't even have to focus on a single page because it's going so fast! But every once in awhile I see a page and I get hooked into it. One lifetime I was a dancing girl in India. And I'm wearing these amazing colors and I'm twirling like a whirling dervish and I have bangles on my ankles and my wrists and I'm twirling in ecstasy; and at that moment the shaman's in front of me, rattling; "State your intention!" I got off the path. "My intention is to ... every lifetime, heal every misperception, and having done that I want to be with God. So now I'm in the misperception phase and I say this 3 times. I focus on ... every time he brings me back. That was amazing; I have no idea how long that was.*

*After that was over I again shoot out of a canon; not a rocket ship; I shoot out of a canon and I am physically experiencing every life form one after another. Starting at that beginning part – and I couldn't control it. But from the moment of my inception as a life form on the planet; I'm experiencing every life form from the tiniest speck of soil, amoebas in water; growing and growing into these various life forms – evolution. And then I'm aware that I can be present in the room at the same time. So I'm plugging into other people's journeys too! I'm like — Alberto is outside. There is a jaguar! And, the jaguar is my power animal! And, he becomes jaguar and he is out there in the jungle and he is roaring and roaring. And, then at one point I hear him; he's sitting next to me; the shaman he's asking for direction in his brain pathways. In Spanish — and I understand enough Spanish to know what he's doing; and I say to myself "oh my he's done this so much he's carving new pathways in his brain! Ginny, be present; be aware! This is your first carving here! So I'm back in my journey and the shaman says, "State your intention…" don't get lost. I get back into my journey. I'm at the place where I state my intention: "I want to be with God!" I've gone to the source of my beginning; I want to be with God. [what did you mean by carving new pathways?] To carve new pathways in the brain for new knowledge.*

*So now I'm going to be with God. All of a sudden I again get shot out of a canon. But I'm not an "I"! I'm not a body! I'm not anything! I do have my breath and now I'm like a giant amoebic — what do call those things — you make a fire — and I can experience the universe as this — deeeeep inhalation, deeeeep exhalation with arms going away from the body and her arms going toward her body — it is me! it's around me! it's the only thing that exists; and then if I could say that a smile comes over my being; it wasn't a physical smile because I wasn't a physical being; the awareness in that moment [sobbing] I was God! I was — [I say: "experiencing the breath of the life force of the universe"] — and there was nothing else! And I was there! So there wasn't any thought, there wasn't anything. And the next thing that I remember was coming back into my physical body and I was sitting in lotus for however long that was.*

*I don't sit in lotus; I don't sit in lotus for long periods. My legs opened up; my eyes were closed; I positioned myself near the wall of the building because I didn't know if I was going to pass out or not. I said to myself, at least you won't pass out on the floor if you're leaning against the wall. I set myself up so I wouldn't fall. So I leaned back and my hands went to my abdomen and my hands were way out! I was 9 months pregnant! And I just — I was sobbing, just sobbing and all of a sudden I was in labor! I said, "oh my god! I'm having a baby!" And I went through labor completely. I birthed a baby! And at the end of this birth I took this deep, deep sigh and said, "oh my god! I birthed myself! And my friend was sitting next to me, staring at me. And she said "I've been with you for the last 2 hours of your journey! Mine was over 2 hours ago. "You just birthed yourself!!" "I witnessed your entire birth!!!" [we are both crying]. And then I looked around the room — the shaman was gone. Alberto was gone! There were only 4 people in the room. Everybody was gone! And we were done."*

A quote from an interview with an educated, well traveled professional man who traveled to the Andes and had a mystic experience engaging in the ritual of San Pedro:

*"After various preparations and ceremonial proceedings, including chanting, rattling, and rattling leaves on my head, we were ready. As I heard the shaman come up behind me as I stood at the mesa [ceremonial altar], he said — drink. And I did. And, there it began. As I sat on the bank of the river [a tributary headwater of the Amazon River] right out front of where we had convened the mesa, I began to feel detached from my body in an odd sort of way. First the detachment was controllable and euphoric and then it became deeply introspective and then universally expansive. There is not such a thing as time. It does not exist, I understood. I found myself delving into the deepest inner expansions of my being cyclically with expansive outward bounds of my consciousness like the breath of life. In and out, only my breath of consciousness brought me into and then out of myself and into all that which we are together. I was nurtured by the energy that I belong to — our universe, us. I saw God, us. We and everything are God, I understood. There I was with no concepts of anything but the exact present. Everything about it, as grand as it is! The breathing in and out became more and more intensified and there I went into a timeless, pressureless, pleasurefull space, it was bliss as I divined my purpose and was spoken to by the divine energies which envelop and make up us all and vice versa. I recall vividly [as we were then moving down a river in a boat] the conversations that I was having with the living river, heavens and the tall majestic tree beings who cradled me in their arms, so beautiful were their smiles and caresses, their flowing hair, lips, faces, they are beautiful and we talked. Not with words you see, but with intention, theirs was known to me and mine to them. Theirs to me was love — mine to them was love, and I have continued on in that stead since.*

An intense altered state of consciousness, a powerful state of mind, is quite evident in the sexual and emotional acts of love; an experience that can transport one into a transformative space. Neurological researchers have demonstrated a strong connection between sexuality and trance. It appears that women have a greater capacity to experience a greater intensity than men.[13] The electrical connections across the hemispheres of a woman's brain contribute to their heightened experience. This is because there is a greater number and higher density of neurons in a woman's brain which connect and coordinate the hemispheres. The *corpus callosum*, the major anatomy that connects and coordinates the hemispheres of the brain, has a greater equality of connection between the two hemispheres and is larger in women than in men. Furthermore, the *anterior commissure*, a neural pathway connecting the two hemispheres of the brain, is larger and denser in women. And, the band of fibers connecting the thalami of the two hemispheres, the *massa intermedia*, is found more often in women than in men.[13]  This provides a woman with a potential for intense orgasms that propel her into an altered state of consciousness culminating in an ecstasy that appears to be similar to indigenous individuals who have been possessed by spirits.  This capacity provides women with extraordinary skills in shamanic practice.  In fact, Barbara Tedlock points out that the word for orgasm is the same as the word for trance in many languages!

It is this great capacity of the human mind, the capacity to access a wide range of experiences from a number of body, and specifically brain sources, that give us our potential for experiencing spirit and achieving spirituality.  These higher levels of consciousness do not arise from our normal everyday routine experiences.  They come from a special learning and a discipline that trains and entrains the mind to emerge into higher levels of consciousness and knowing.  This realm of knowledge and consciousness is necessary for the healthful survival of culture, society, and the individuals who are a part of that society.  It is normally the elders of traditional society, men and women who have experienced the joys and excitements, the sadness and tragedy, the challenges and tribulations of life, who are the teachers for the younger members of a community.  In modern urban societies, the culture of science and technology, corporate business and media advertizing, has taken over the governance of the culture and the programming of uncritical individual minds.  The wisdom of our teachers has been eclipsed by the culture of materialism, individualism, and narcissism and has led to a whole host of ills — medical, nutritional, psychological, economic, and political — ills that crept into the space left vacant by the traditional wisdom of the elders who lived connected to nature and cosmos, valued the quality of intimacy in relationships, and knew how to experience joy in everyday life.  Thus, it is in the next chapter that we learn about that higher level of consciousness that enables the individual to experience a greater peace of mind, lessen the possibility of afflictions, and heighten the possibility of teaching the knowledge to a younger generation.

# Chapter 5
## Spirit: Cultivating Consciousness

*"The idea of a universal mind or Logos would be, I think, a fairly plausible inference from the present state of scientific theory."*

**Arthur Eddington**

*"Let us learn to dream, gentlemen; then we shall perhaps find the truth."*

**Friedrich Kekule**

*"Here I am, behold me... I am the Sun behold me... "*

**Lakota Prayer**

*"The wonderful host of rays has risen: the eye of Mitra, Varuna, and Agni: the Sun, the soul of all that moves or Immovable, has filled the heaven, the Earth and the firmament."*

**Rig Veda**

*"One of the gods, Quetzalcoatl, faced the east, and there, off in the distance, the sun rose just over the horizon."*

**Popol Vuh**

This concept, "spirit", has a multitude of meanings and varies in the minds of individuals contingent on their momentary orientation and cultural learning. In the American English lexicon there are greater than 20 meanings to this term.[1,2] These meanings refer to the animating principle of life or vital essence; the soul; the incorporeal aspect of humans; supernatural beings; an attitude or principle that pervades a thought; the source of feelings that prompts action; temperament or disposition; and even fermented beverages to name several. For our purposes in this chapter, we focus on the concept of spirit as it relates to spirituality, referring to a very special human quality revered in cultures around the world. It is a state of being conferring a quality of life widely recognized and admired, yet achieved by a relative few. But in every population of our world spiritual people exist, in groups or in solitude.

The qualities of spirituality represent the ideal qualities of the human condition as they stand for peace, happiness and fulfillment. Thus spirituality represents a positive direction in the evolution of our species contingent on an increasing number of people's orientation and actualization of these qualities and life ways.

Evidence from the ethnographic record and data from a variety of disciplines, including archaeology, anthropology, psychology, gerontology, philosophy, health sciences, and evolutionary biology, suggest a way of life that creates new possibilities for the human condition and the environment we inhabit through spirituality. That environment is one of a grounded environment that respects the laws and principles of evolution, nature, and survival in a global community. That state of being in the world that promises higher levels of consciousness is spirituality—in the multitude of expressions that manifest among human beings. We will point out in this chapter that not only the recognized universal personal qualities of spirituality are relevant here; we find that the ideal characteristics of the healer across cultures (of oneself, of others, of their respective communities, of earth, and of the environment) on the road to wellness, recent research findings on happiness, the conditions of longevity, and environmental interconnectedness all dovetail and reinforce one another creating a synergy of maximized vitality and high human potential. An evolutionary perspective on these various qualities suggests an orientation and direction for citizens of the human species to consider in their contributions to a new world order—one of heightened consciousness. In contrast to the ideal characteristics of people and environment it is useful to briefly consider those conditions that have created the antithesis—states of conflict and violence, unhappiness, and lack of fulfillment at all levels of social and cultural complexity.

Spirituality is about connecting to and grounding through nature, what we have always done throughout our diverse journey through humanity, and before. It describes an inward journey of exploration which ultimately takes us outward and expansively into the cosmos and all that is and has ever been. It is embodied by potentiation and actualization, our latent abilities, and marks our journey toward understanding.

At the dawn of sapienization, and very possibly before, we were endowed with certain abilities, capacities and potentials that soared beyond normal personality structure. These capabilities are still observable today among certain "gifted" individuals across many if not all populations. Since these potentials vary in amongst individuals, those who can articulate and communicate their gifts are very often seen as teachers, gurus, and spiritual leaders. These potentials are expressed as psychic phenomena including telepathy, remote viewing, precognition, psychokinesis, out of body experiences, existence in the pure present, ability to see through the illusion of linear time, and ability to see through the illusion of individuality. These phenomena, in large part, have been scientifically documented.[3]

In order to appreciate that these abilities became buried throughout our course of evolution, one must realize that when the newer regions of the brain evolved, the more primitive regions of the brain became less active. But these latent abilities can become more activated in ritual, cleansing, fasting, ceremony, trance states, and dreamtime to name a few.[3]

Dreamtime, or REM sleep (named for the rapid eye movements that occur in this sleep stage) is one aspect of these latent abilities which we have all experienced to varying degrees. While it is widely speculated that dreamtime serves various functions including learning, processing of emotional content or even accessing higher realms of being, it is clear that our ancestors governed themselves in part based on dreamtime. Indeed, the ancient Egyptians built huge temples for the induction of prophetic dreams and Australian Aborigines believe that knowledge is first acquired during dreamtime[3] — just two examples of what was commonplace throughout the diverse human experience. It is likely that the evolution of REM sleep occurred between 130 and 210 million years ago.[3] This is well before the expanding neocortex and frontal lobes occurred in our *H. erectus* (1.9 million years ago) to *H. sapien* (0.5 million years ago) ancestors.[3] It is these regions of the brain which enable cognition and linear thought. These regions enable goals, orientation and forward thinking. They also enable chatter and neurotic thought such as: What about this? What about that? Should I do this? Should I do that? What if I had done this? What if I had done that? These latter-developed regions, in essence, divert our consciousness of the present moment by dwelling in the past and future. When these regions are quieted, more primitive regions are potentiated enabling heightened consciousness. It has since been scientifically demonstrated that our latent abilities are less fragmentary in dreamtime.[3] And, the objective of meditation and the Yoga mind are the quieting of these regions which prevent complete presence and unbounded consciousness.

Throughout humanity, there are individuals, both men and women, oftentimes considered "gifted" who stand out in the community and occupy the roles of diviner, healer, mediator, fortune-teller, story-teller, and teacher. These individuals most often are normal citizens of their communities making a living by conventional occupations, yet performing their exceptional roles when members of the community appealed to them. We most often recognize them as spiritual people, or, as shamans who reach out into hyperspace[4] to receive information that may ameliorate a condition, be it medical, personal, social or environmental. The shaman mobilizes supernormal powers with the aid of a spiritual technology requiring the performance of ritual, the expression of love, and the establishment of grounding to name a few. This technology includes drums, rattles, music, chanting, entheogens, and the like—to be discussed in fuller detail elsewhere in this work.

## An Evolutionary Perspective on Vitality and Aging: Steps Toward Spirituality

Almost two million years ago our *H. erectus* ancestors were already crossing the threshold toward humanity. The problems of adaptive survival were being worked out. In the works was a burgeoning cognitive brain and a family-based social structure. Life expectancy was roughly 35 – 45 years. These beings had a great vulnerability to climate, accident, disease, and unexpected death; these issues were very real, palpable, and omnipresent.

The heightening instincts of social life and creative communication allowed for an emotional sensitivity to the exigencies, joys, and sorrows of daily life. In this context we speculate that a nucleus of emotionality evolved along with the neocortex. A configuration of emotion included fear, love, hope, the plea, and faith or belief, emerging as a configuration that became a gestalt for the nurturing of humanizing culture. The singularity of these separate emotional states became galvanized and transformed in the context of ultimate concerns, the penultimate of which was the realization of the *inevitability* of death. This synthesis of emotional states within the body of ultimate concerns emerged as a cultural revolution, giving birth to spirituality which provided mystical explanations to inscrutable questions. These explanations were based upon preexisting primordial sentiments and capabilities, grounded in nature.

Some of the "glue" that held people together in community was the natural world, commonly shared tethers, and the empathic sense, defined as the capacity to cognitively and emotionally understand the experience of another. The capacity for empathy lives in potentiation but must be learned and developed as a skill to be practiced within family and community. Based on this newly evolved cognition and the preexisting primordial sentiments the nuclear family and the 3-generation extended family became institutionalized.

Oftentimes, our elder-teachers are spiritual people, grounded in the balance of nature and sense of the ideals of humanity. As we developed our humanity and civilization our longevity increased. It is our position, however, that our true longevity potential is not realized, but a shadow of this potential currently exists. For example, longevity declined with the industrial era, pollution and close living under unhygienic conditions. Once these burdens were ameliorated (basic hygiene, for example) it once again rose.  Our longevity is currently going down[5] due to stress related illness and diseases of civilization—we need to remedy this.

It is normally around middle age that the capacity for the empathic experience becomes most salient, if it is developed at all, in a particular individual.  Women have this capacity to a larger extent and at a younger age.  It is at middle age that a sobriety and maturity about life normally develops.  And, from the insight into one's mortality one may develop a personal spirituality or even a religiosity, given already in one's culture and encouraged by one's knowledge of one's limited time on earth.  Now, what we call mid-life was that very same time that normatively, was the end of life for persons in considerable portions of earlier eras.

Through language and culture the human species proved unique in having evolved an open system of growth and social and personal development.  Aging after mid-life signals a new challenge for members of society.  The social challenge is to learn or relearn the roles of grand-parenting and elderhood in community.  The personal challenge is to remain healthy and joyful and a valued asset to family and community.

Aging after mid-life offers the challenge of recouping and rediscovering those human attributes that allowed our survival and growth and societal development from the very beginning.  These attributes are the very qualities found in childhood, for human beings are truly neotenous beings, having the capacity to retain those qualities developed in childhood.[6]

The wisdom of accumulated human experience inclines one, if not obligates one, to teach the basic lessons of life.  In tribal society this is accomplished through song, poetry, story-telling, mythology, and oral history.  It is through these traditions that love is mobilized and the art of loving is learned in human encounters.  It is also important to note here that the elders provide a connection to the next generation through this inter-generational transmission of knowledge.

Because grand-parents and aging adults are free from the primary responsibility of the discipline of children and the emotional conflicts engendered therein, they are fit for being the best teachers of their grandchildren.  Timeless traditions have shown grandparents to be the childcare providers, the music, dance, and sex educators, and the story-tellers that instill a sense of history and identity in their grandchildren.  Aging adults are the best emotional educators.  They can disseminate important information as living examples of what life holds for all throughout the lifecycle. They are the nurturers of the young, providing information, value, and culture. They are the "nurturing means through which the wealth of humanity is realized in the fulfillment of the unique potentialities of each of society's members".[6]

## Personal Qualities of Spirituality

We often find that spirituality and religion are tied together, but we also recognize that spirituality transcends any particular religion and can reference ones particular journey to understanding, which may or may not involve religion.

Spirituality can be taken to mean many things to many people. For example, it could be conceived as a "state of being" which William James asserts and, as discussed in Moro et al, 2008,[4] James maintains that this state of being is universal. It involves a group of spiritual emotions that form the "habitual center" of personal energy. This habitual center includes a feeling of being in a wider life than that of the world's selfish interests, a direct conviction of the existence of an higher power, a sense of the friendly continuity of this power with our life and a willing self-surrender to its control, a feeling of elation and freedom resulting from the escape from confining selfhood, a shifting of the center of emotions toward loving and harmonious affections, a move toward yes and away from no.[6]

Spirituality is consistent, stable, and grounding. There is an inner consistency which is manifest as a permanent set of values. And "there is an awareness of the presence of the power that some religions call "God" and this awareness is a source of repose and confidence".[6]

Let us compare the realms of science, religion, and spirituality: science is the realm of empirically based knowing; religion is the realm of believing or "faith"; spirituality is the realm of being. The aim of the spiritual life is to raise the level of being and consciousness of the engaged person; to understand the meaning of life in terms of direct personal experience. The fruits of this expansion of consciousness include an indifference to possessions; capacity for impartial, objective love, capacity for compassion, indifference to physical discomfort, complete freedom from the fear of death; charity is the greatest fruit of the spiritual life and the concept of "Bodhisattva" (regarding sentient beings with compassion) has the same emphasis on charity.[6]

## Attributes of the Healer: Spiritual Personification

We suggest here that the attributes of the healer conflate and complement those qualities we recognize as spiritual—spiritual people are healers and healers are spiritual people. We believe the healer, along with midwifery and tool-making, are some of the oldest of professions reaching back before full humanization.

The healer stands alone as a special kind of person. The role of the healer is universal, found in all societies and cultures of the world. We prefer to think of these practitioners on a skill or effectiveness-based continuum rather than a dichotomy of practitioner vs. non-practitioner. Just as we find great medical doctors, acceptable medical doctors, and poor medical doctors (regardless of their credentials), we can conceive of particular healers on a gradient of effectiveness in terms of their influence on their patients and community as well as their effectiveness with maintaining their own level of spirituality. Carl Rogers suggested three critical qualities necessary for effective therapy, in his case, psychotherapy: congruence including genuineness and personality integration; unconditional positive regard including warm acceptance and non-possessive caring; and empathy: understanding the client's experience correctly.

Additional research has shown that effective healers are also intelligent, responsible, creative, sincere, energetic, warm, tolerant, respectful, supportive, self-confident, keenly attentive, benign, concerned, reassuring, firm, persuasive, encouraging, credible, sensitive, gentle, and trustworthy. These traits may not all be universal—but we can consider them as ideal qualities. Furthermore, each trait may be conceptualized on a continuum both synchronically and diachronically. That is, healers may be placed on a continuum for each trait from nonexistent, poor, through to highly successful. And a particular trait of a specific healer may place differently on this continuum from day to day depending on one's social situation, mood, client specifics and difficulty of the condition addressed. Nevertheless, on an ideal plane, we can consider these traits convincingly important in the treatment of clients and community and environment. We may also keep in mind that these traits may be highly beneficial to the person who possesses them and the community that learns from them.

## Spirituality and Happiness

Are spiritual people and healers happy? There has been a growing interest and research in wellness and happiness in recent years. This interest is seen in the authors from a number of disciplines who have contributed to the subject. The *Journal of Happiness Studies: An Interdisciplinary Forum On Subjective Well-Being*, edited by R. Cummins, provides an outlet for this kind of research. A notable author on the subject is psychologist Sonja Lyubomirsky, Ph.D., Stanford University, who explains why the study of happiness and well-being is important in human research:

*"In short, because most people believe happiness is meaningful, desirable, and an important worthy goal, because happiness is one of the most salient and significant dimensions of human experience and emotional life, because happiness yields numerous rewards for the individual, and because it makes for a better, healthier, stronger society."*

Dr. Lyubomirsky's years of research has shown that chronically happy and unhappy persons are systematically different and normally conduct their lives cognitively and motivationally in a manner that supports their respective dispositions.

Are there benefits to being happy? Continuing research clearly reveals the implications for society synchronically as well as diachronically over both short periods of time and extended periods of time, which also spells out the implications for human evolution.

*"A recent review of all the available literature has revealed that happiness does indeed have numerous positive byproducts, which appear to benefit not only individuals, but families, communities, and the society at large. The benefits of happiness include higher income and superior work outcomes (e.g., more satisfying and longer marriages, more friends, stronger social support, and richer social interactions), more activity, energy, and flow, and better physical health (e.g., a bolstered immune system, lowered stress levels, and less pain) and even longer life."*

From their focus groups and studies and analyses of their case protocols Rick Foster and Greg Hicks have come up with a most interesting book, *How We Choose to be Happy.*[7] They define happiness as:

*"...a profound, enduring feeling of contentment, capability and centeredness. It's a rich sense of well-being that comes from knowing you can deal productively and creatively with all that life offers – both the good and the bad. It's knowing your internal self and responding to your real needs, rather than the demands of others. And it's a deep sense of engagement – living in the moment and enjoying life's bounty."*

Their nine parameters of happiness[7] are:

1. Intention: the active desire and commitment to be happy and the fully conscious decision to choose happiness over unhappiness.

2. Accountability: the choice to create the life you want to live, to assume full personal responsibility for your actions, thoughts and feelings, and the emphatic refusal to blame others for your own unhappiness.

3. Identification: the ongoing process of looking deeply within yourself to assess what makes you uniquely happy, apart from what you're told by others should make you happy.

4. Centrality: the nonnegotiable insistence on making that which creates happiness central in your life.

5. Recasting: the choice to convert problems into opportunities and challenges and to transform trauma into something meaningful, important and a source of emotional energy.

6. Options: the decision to approach life by creating multiple scenarios, to be open to new possibilities and to adopt a flexible approach to life's journey.

7. Appreciation: the choice to appreciate deeply your life and the people in it and to stay in the present by turning each experience into something precious.

8. Giving: the choice to share yourself with friends and community and to give to the world at large without the expectation of a "return".

9. Truthfulness: the choice to be honest with yourself and others in an accountable manner by not allowing societal, corporate or family demands to violate your internal contract.

## Impediments to Happiness and thus Wellbeing

The authors Foster and Hicks[7] also suggest thirty-five ego defenses that may act as barriers to happiness. A sample of these are given here: loss of humor, taking offense, playing dumb, being highly critical and needing to be right, wanting the last word, flooding with information to prove a point, endless explaining and rationalizing, playing the victim, rigidity—"I'm not willing to change", denial, withdrawal into silence, cynicism and sarcasm, confusion, eccentricity, being too nice, holding a grudge, inappropriate laughter, self-deprecation.

## Transformational Processes

Reminick[8] has proposed a relative deprivation macro-model of motivation. The first part deals with the causes of discontent that he asserts account for a great deal of psychosocial phenomena from stress-related illness to mass violence.[9] The second part deals with culturally determined modalities for the transformation of potentially destructive energy into socially productive and creative behavior.

He begins with a deprivation-derived model of motivation. As Abraham Maslow said long ago, a satisfied need is no longer a motivation. Reminick's model is a causal chain which is a sequence of dispositions that begins with a state of deprivation leading to other stage-related dispositional responses:

*Deprivation>Frustration>Hostility>Aggression>Modes of Response*

Each of these successive states may be conceived as a continuum of emotional energy, from weak to strong, determined by the nature and strength of the stimulus, the life history of an individual, and the character and mental structure of that individual.

Needs are either innate or derived. Deprivations create needs. For simplification we can posit a dichotomy of deprivations: absolute and relative. Absolute deprivations refer to basic needs for food, shelter, protection, nurturance, touch, cognitive stimulation, and the like. Traumatic experience at this level can engender long-lasting psychological infirmities which can manifest mentally, physically or spiritually.

Relative deprivation develops when feelings of frustration are aroused because one's situation does not meet one's expectations or desires. The basic categories of relative deprivation, as Aberle[9] suggested, are possessions, status, self worth, behavior, and power. These represent basic needs which are shaped by the culture in terms of the ideals and expectations of that culture. Reminick suggests that the closer one gets to one's goal the higher the motivation and the nearer the barrier to the goal the higher the frustration and the greater the sense of deprivation because of the a) nearness of the goal, and b) the amount of investment along the path across the barriers to the goal.

The anger, either conscious or unconscious, leads to certain dispositional modes of response. The first 5 response categories are fairly primitive: *impulsivity* or lashing out, *displacement, involution,* i.e., emotional depression or psychosomatic response such as sudden ailments or afflictions, *social isolation,* and *denial.* The sixth category involves creative responses to these deprivations or unfulfilled needs. In most cases culture provides modalities for the shaping and expression of the energy needed in the investment. This includes all varieties of sports or athletic contests and competitions, rituals, milestones, verbal contests, law and order, literature, poetry, art, medicine, military, police or other authority, social movements, and lastly, for our purposes, spirituality and spiritual movements. The last categories are normally initiated with the recognition of *anomie* and the search for a greater meaning in one's life. The sources of deprivation are many and the options for alleviating the frustrations are many, positive channels must be sought after understanding deprivations.

## Revitalization

When a cohort of the population realizes that they are unhappy or deprived on some levels, and that there is another, more satisfying way of life to welcome and the communication of this way of life reaches a "critical mass" they are ready for change. The first stage of this change is for that cohort, early adopters, of the population to recognize the leaders and teachers of that change. This often requires an intelligent charismatic personality who can communicate and reflect the ills of a people and offer a path to a more satisfying way of life. In America, the Black Nationalist movement led by Elijah Mohammad and the Black human rights movement led by Malcolm X; and the Civil Rights movement led by Dr. Martin Luther King are good examples of revitalization movements with spiritual elements. In the contemporary world there is nature as a teacher, and there are many other teachers and charismatic personalities from many walks of life including yogis, new age shamans, psychologists, ecologists and environmentalists, physicians, nutritionists, cosmologists, psychics, people who offer stress relief and show the way to happiness, and importantly traditionalists and elders. This sets in motion a process that Wallace[10] termed "revitalization movements" which appear to be universal and sporadically occurring in the various parts of the world since time immemorial.

Wallace's paradigm of 6 phases are not mutually exclusive. The initiation of successive phases may include the previous phases and operate simultaneously and reinforce one another. Then, as the earlier phases wane in response to the gaining momentum of the later phases, the movement approaches maturity.

The first phase of the movement is the *formulation of a code* where the intelligencia of the movement articulates the issues of the masses and articulates a pathway to a better life.

The second phase is *communication*. The ideology must be communicated; must be preached and evangelized through personal communication and the media. This communication must accomplish several goals: It must articulate the problem of the people; it must mobilize the sentiments of those involved; it must articulate the nature of the deprivations; and it must offer a way out of the commonly experienced problems. The communication must also offer both material, social, and spiritual rewards that is expressed as a "superior way of life".

The third phase is *organization*. This phase is what we call the "politicization of discontent". The cohort of the population must realize their discontent and mobilize for change both on personal and social levels. They must access the avenues to political power to assist them in actualizing their goals. The leader must recognize his or her disciples and these people must create an organization to communicate, fund, recruit, and legitimate their movement.

The fourth phase is *adaptation*. At this stage there is both an internal and external challenge. The movement most certainly adapts to the sociopolitical environment of the larger society yet keeps from being perceived as a threat to that society. Furthermore, the movement must adapt to the internal strains, conflicts, factions, and inadequacies and maintain internal integrity and development.

The fifth phase of the revitalization movement is *cultural transformation* which signals the transformation of a significant part of society to a new way of life; a way of life that is self-fulfilling and sustainable and can be offered to the next generation. It is the stage of "organizational maturity and efficacy".[10]

The final phase of this process is *routinization* when pattern stability is achieved and the various aspects of the ideology, values, and social agencies become institutionalized.[10,11]

## Architecture of Spirituality and Wellbeing

On an institutional level, government must support an ecology that cares for the people and encourages a balance of nature, the promotion of spirituality, and the cultivation of consciousness while frustrating the narcissism and greed of the oligarchy. This involves community leaders who are knowledgeable about the healthy living of humans, animals and plant life and serve the principles of the balance of nature and who maintain the priority of ecology over the convenience of jobs or other economic motives.

Government must facilitate educational institutions whose members teach healthy living, promote mind-building creative (not only literary) mentalities, including music, recreation and creativity of individual students; where school food places serve items that help brains grow and eliminate those items that contribute to the mental and social ills of youth, viz., sugar, the dangerous high fructose corn syrup, unhealthy fats, preservatives, toxic dyes, and caffeine. On this same governmental level we must expand our federally-funded parent agencies that provide information for informed living and healthy childrearing. On this institutional level religious institutions must recognize and promote their grounding in nature, teach the qualities of spirituality and profess the balance of powers of the universe.

The State University of New York (SUNY) presented international spiritual leader and humanitarian of notable stature Sri Mata Amritananda Mayi Devi (Amma) with an honorary doctorate in humane letters on May 25, 2010. They did so in recognition of her efforts in global peace, education, and the far-reaching impact of her charitable organizations in relieving poverty and human suffering in India and internationally. SUNY president John B. Simpson said, "Through this conferral, we pay tribute to the far-reaching contributions of a distinguished educational leader, prominent humanitarian and esteemed spiritual leader. Through her leadership of Amrita University as well as through her humanitarian work, Chancellor Amma exemplifies the value of international dialogue and dedicated public service in the global arena. These are values at the core of the University at Buffalo's mission as an internationalized public university seeking to prepare our students to contribute meaningfully to the global world." Amma delivered an address focused on education in which she discussed the importance of the inclusion of 1) universal spiritual values in core curricula, 2) the role of meditation in developing and gaining control over the mind, and 3) the complementary relationships between scientific knowledge and spiritual wisdom. She said, "It is Amma's prayer that we develop the expansive-mindedness to embrace both scientific knowledge and spiritual wisdom. We can no longer afford to see these two streams of knowledge as flowing in opposite directions. In truth, they complement one another. If we merge these streams, we will find that we are able to create a mighty river—a river whose waters can remove suffering and spread life to all of humanity."

On the level of individual wellbeing there must be a sense of mission and calling, vision and commitment. One's work must excite with the expectation of fulfillment.

One can create an identity around the mission in one's life. Satellite activities in life should be built around and be in conjunction with the mission.

## Our Revolutionary Crest: Heightened Consciousness

Cultural Creatives, a term coined by sociologist Paul Ray and psychologist Sherry Ruth Anderson, after greater than 13 years of survey research studies on over 100,000 Americans, plus over 100 focus groups and dozens of in-depth interviews,[12] describes a large segment in Western society that has recently emerged outside of the standard paradigm of Modernist vs Traditionalist. They presented their findings in their book published in 2000 called *The Cultural Creatives: How 50 Million People are Changing the World.*[12] Essentially, Cultural Creatives care deeply about nature, ecology, sustainability, wholesome relationships, holistic health, world peace, and social justice and they value altruism, self actualization and expression, and spirituality.

It is the Cultural Creative demographic which spawned and drives the Lifestyles of Health and Sustainability (LOHAS) market which describes an estimated $209 billion U.S. marketplace for goods and services focused on holistic health, sustainable environment, social justice issues, personal/spiritual development and sustainable life ways for all.13 LOHAS consumers represent approximately 19% percent of the adults in the U.S. They purchase fair-trade, organic, and sustainable goods.13 In effect, they are committed to socially responsible consumption for people and planet. This market force represents our evolution and heightened consciousness. This is a revitalization movement.

## Conclusion: Cultivating Consciousness via Spirituality

We maintain that spirituality is about connecting to and grounding through nature, it is about an inward journey which takes us outward into the cosmos and all that is, and it is potentiation and actualization of latent abilities in us all — our journey toward understanding, the cultivation of consciousness toward peace, happiness and fulfillment.

# Chapter 6
# The Good Life: An Architecture for Holistic Health and Wellness

*"Drink your tea slowly and reverently, as if this activity is the axis on which the whole earth revolves. Live the moment. Only this actual moment is life."*

**Thich Nhat Hanh**

*"Nature is not only stranger than we suppose, it is stranger than we can suppose."*

**J. B. S. Haldane**

*"When the mind has settled, we are established in our essential nature, which is unbounded consciousness. Our essential nature is usually overshadowed by the activity of the mind."*

**Yoga Sutras of Patanjali**

The Good Life is achieved by one's awareness and practice of holistic health. This cannot be achieved until one's consciousness extends to the variety and levels of environments that influence our lives, seen diachronically, as environments change through time, and synchronically, as it exists today, for better or worse. The Good Life entails accessing resources that satisfy the basic needs of human beings, that maintains horizons of biological, psychological, and spiritual growth, creating strong, healthy communities that provide the opportunities to maximize one's natural potentials. This can only happen within a healthy environment. This environment is not only the natural physical environment we live in but also the environment of beautiful communities, the environment of healthy individuals who enjoy their vitality, who nurture the environment of their very cells, all one hundred trillion plus of them, including the energy of our aura fields which emanate from our bodies and connect us to each other and all that is around us.

The World Health Organization defines health as a state of complete physical, mental and social wellbeing and not merely the absence of disease or infirmity.[1] Our work contributes the concept of holism to this definition and promotes recognition of our inextricable, interdependence to everything around us. This journey to wellness, or understanding and application of health, certainly involves an appreciation of complex interplay of systems in balance and includes constructs of the mind, body, spirit and environment, both social and natural worlds.[2] Our aim is to appreciate this interdependence of living systems and to understand the conditions that maintain it and know the threats to it. We also recognize that we face a number of serious and very complex problems in health and wellness on both local and global levels. One thing is for certain, it is easier and cheaper to prevent disease than to treat it. It is a poor strategy and unsustainable to continue to apply elaborate technological interventions for modern human afflictions. Traditional knowledge and social responsibility will take us a long way to achieving our ideals and removing the threats to our environments and ourselves.

Health, wellness and their inextricable linkage to nature and our environment are not given nearly the attention that they merit. Our complex ecologies and our unique niche in our ecosystem are all but ignored by modern healthcare, media bought by vested interests, business and industry putting profit over human welfare, and educational institutions that promote literacy and not creativity while proffering unhealthy food to our children. The general public is largely ignorant of the inimical influences in their lives. For example, the epidemic of childhood and adult obesity and the high incidence of diabetes in the U.S. is due, in large part, to the ingestion of high fructose corn syrup; and add to this the overconsumption of other varieties of sugars, fats, and caffeine. Attention to how one fits into the environment, i.e., the ecological factor is largely ignored. This condition is exacerbated by the disconnection from our environment, without which we do not survive. How are we to expect our children to understand and appreciate the beauty and wonderment of the forest if they do not or cannot experience it? It is the responsibility and the privilege and the honor of parents to teach their children!

Without pure water, clean air, and nutritious food, we cannot attain health. It is impossible to detoxify while ingesting toxic-laden water and food. It is impossible to be nutritionally complete from depleted soils, air, and waters; and all of this is dependent upon the sustained health of our ecosystems and indeed our planet Earth.

A sustainable health and wellness indicator could involve a fundamental connection of the growth of economic metrics such as *Gross Domestic Product* "GDP" with the sustained availability of our natural resources and the overall health and wellness of the people which the GDP serves. We would do well to reverse the social and economic trends toward continued investment in the infirmity of the population. We must continue to seek more sustainable means toward attaining health and wellness. A holistic approach, one which unites our economy with our ecology and in a fashion that promotes a nurturing, healthful environment is essential and should be our global priority. This holistic approach would include holistic constructs involving mental, physical, spiritual and environmental health viability.[2]

One strategy which brings great possibility in effective, sustainable wellness is holistic health promotion; in effect, learning from traditions and the integration of successful, adaptable traditional health practices into mainstream healthcare.[3,4,5,6] We can, and must, learn from our traditions, from the elders who taught from the wisdom of their experience and from our modern teachers who teach from the wisdom of traditional peoples around the world.

Throughout much of the last century, longevity has been increasing, however, recently this trend has been reversing in the developed world likely due to diseases of civilization and stress related illness among others.[7] Further, we do not know exactly what our natural longevity should be, certainly there have been a multitude of centenarians throughout the millennia, we investigate their secrets of long life through their contemporary counterparts and highlight them in this work. We do so to illustrate our new possibilities in health from learning from traditional practices since it seems that though technology is a new tool, it is not solving our heath problems and at times it is even adding to them. While more and more people are accelerating into the elder demographic the quality of life these people experience appears to decline with their age as seen in our out-of-control "health-care" meaning, disease care, statistics. As an example, in 2006, there were approximately 37 million people living in the U.S. who were 65 or older, representing approximately 12 percent of the population. Projected estimates suggest that by 2030 there will be approximately 72 million people living in the U.S. who will be 65 and older, representing nearly 20 percent of the total U.S. population.[7] With these aging demographics comes increasing need for effective, affordable, sustainable health and wellness practices—longevity and vital living!

In searching for lifestyles that enhance vitality, longevity and promote the Good Life, the authors have spent collectively the greater part of a century looking into traditional health and wellness practices the world over as exemplified by longest-lived cultures and people. For it is they from whom we can learn. They express a positive attitude that is essential to long life and the Good Life. Adding life to years rather than adding years to life is the goal to which these elders strive. They understand that health and balance of mind, body, and spirit in the context of a nurturing environment is essential to our health and wellbeing. They point out, in their many languages, that intimacy and connection with nature is of primary importance. Striving to lead a stress-free life is very much a part of their day-to-day routine and practice. They tend to work toward living in the present, as such they don't dwell on the past too much, nor do they spend too much time focusing in the future. There is a belief that one's consciousness of the present provides abundance for the future. For this they are grateful to be able to experience the present as it is. This notion is widely expressed in the Eastern philosophies. These elders do not live within a fear-based disposition. They exhibit an aura of optimism and sense of humor and lightheartedness in conversation and action. This is apparent in verbal and non-verbal communication with people around them. They are always smiling. And, it is more or less expected that others around them also project the same expression of outward happiness and gratitude for what is. They are quite happy with their life and are hopeful about the future. Misfortune, such as death or illness of loved ones, personal illness, or financial difficulties — these elders show resiliency. They bounce back from difficult situations and learn from them, seeing them as life's processes in a transcendental way. They may even feel gratitude, seeing an unfortunate situation as a learning experience, and work to instill this quality in others with whom they associate. If they come across people who are pessimistic in their outlook, they work to steer them to positive ways of thinking. If they are not successful, they tend to avoid them in a nonspecific pattern of exclusion from close social networks. They assert that staying young and living the Good Life has a lot to do with independence of lifestyle. They do not want to be dependent on others. Every day they wake up in the morning with a new set of jobs to tackle and goals to fulfill.

These healthful and vibrant elders are appreciative of and engaged in cycles of life and what lies beyond. They are not held "captive" to these cycles nor do they adhere in an unquestioning way, but rather are prone to negotiate social forces according to their system of cosmology and ritual. They do not fear death, but embrace it as they embrace the rest of life.

Ritual plays a major role in life. For example, even before a baby is born, the Indian family and community members get involved in the wellbeing and ushering in of the new being. Community responsibility, instead of individual responsibility, in raising the child becomes apparent. Senior-most members of the community play important ritual roles in the practices of their communities. Traditional age-defined roles of the family are observed and respected.

Grandparents fulfill vital roles and functions in their communities. The grandparent role is one of the factors of human survival. Childcare is a critical role within the extended family. It allows the parents to go on with their work, in the home, office, fields and forest.

Grandparents are both the cognitive and emotional teachers of their grandchildren and other youngsters in the community. They supplement the government schools with the traditional ways including music and dance, heritage and history, sexual education, and domestic work roles. It is in the leisure time of the woman and men who have the time and space to perform these critical roles as has been carried out for better then five hundred generations. These are the teachers of aging as well, for the younger members of the community see the behavior and roles that they will eventually assume. The love, reverence, and respect given elders bind them together into a multigenerational solidarity.

The emotional charge often evident between parents and children, because of authority and discipline, is not normally present with the alternate generations. The generation of grandparents can teach the adaptive strategies in navigating through life crises and the conditions of everyday living, across the plateaux of one's maturational stages. These elders inculcate a sense of heritage, of family, lineage, village, and state. This happens through the very powerful modality of story-telling, mythologizing, folk-philosophizing, and casual conversations, often around the hearth fire or on a walk in the woods, valued times with the elders. They learn not only the cognitive history, but, more importantly, the emotional meaning of their history and, consequently, their identity. The elders are the repositories of this knowledge and the benefactors of this history.

A great deal of emotional tension can be generated in normal domestic situations. The elder can be a neutral party with transcendent wisdom that can mediate an emotionally charged conflict. From this grows the mutual support of the transgenerational family and community which then offers this support to its members in a way that does not violate the integrity of the persons involved. Without meaningful mediation the "solutions" attempted can result in confrontations or hostilities.

Feeling comfortable and friendly with others, including strangers is a hallmark of older people, especially, as we have found, the centenarians. They do not fear the opinions of others or how others see them because they have developed their own sense of integrity, authority, authenticity, and identity. They feel comfortable socializing with people of different age groups. They try to keep up to date on what is happening locally, nationally and internationally as best they can. They are willing to learn new things. For example, one Indian elder centenarian on her 106th birthday, registered to learn computer skills at a local school. Interacting with children and teenagers, by telling them oral histories and participating in outdoor activities, are integral parts of their lifestyles. They are willing to express their feelings very freely and openly to others. They take responsibility and care for others when it was within their power. They have aspirations and are comfortable meeting or not meeting them. They appreciate the countryside and the natural resources that sustain them. They live with moral principles—without infringement on the rights of others. They have humility and a tolerance for those who don't have this quality. They love the members of their family and friends who they trust. They allow themselves simple pleasures without the burden of guilt. They teach their ways to the next generation through time spent and by example.

Our longest-lived elders, are predominantly vegetarian or eat diets high in plant products and whole foods and low in animal products. They consume a multitude of freshly picked herbs, vegetables and fruits. The majority of their caloric intake is from fresh, raw vegetables. Sprouted items are common in their diets. They can easily identify herbs, vegetables and fruits with rejuvenating, healing qualities and they consume them regularly. They seldom eat refrigerated items, or foods laden with refined white flour, refined white sugar, preservatives, hydrogenated oils or processed foods of any kind. Their foodstuff is organic in the truest sense of the word grown in areas high in ecological integrity, with nutrient rich soil and virtually devoid of chemical fertilizers, pesticides or herbicides. Every day they eat at the same time, regularly and in small proportions, no one is able to tempt them with larger portions, even if it is their favorite. By Western standards, their daily caloric intake would be considered sparse. However, their calorie-sparse foods are nutrient rich given their predominant fresh, raw, whole foods nature.

They do not involve themselves in lengthy, serious conversation while eating. Eating slowly and concentrating is a part of their routine. For instance, one Indian said "each time you put food in the mouth we need to chew it thirty two times, once for each tooth." They consume large quantities of pure, fresh water, most often from local springs or pristine flowing water right from the earth. Their beverages are not commonly chilled, and are consumed often as teas, or in India, warm water with cumin seeds. They do not drink while they eat, only rarely and if then sparingly. They maintain optimal hydration throughout the day.  Several types of herbs and spices are a regular part of their diet.  Even if they need to travel to other places, they insist on eating at their regular times.  They make it a point not to sleep or lie down at least two hours after they eat.  Fasting is an integral part of their dietary patterns.  Their practices vary mainly from one day per week to two weeks per year.  And, if they imbibe in alcoholic beverages they do so with moderation.  Fermented and cultured beverages are common.

Elders across all cultures and socioeconomic strata, from the time they get up in the morning until they are ready to sleep, are constantly involved in some form of physical or mental activity or purposeful rejuvenating inactivity.  They keep themselves physically and mentally occupied at all times.  They do not call anything "boring" in their daily routines.  And, you will not observe them sitting in one place for an extended period of time, unless it is purposeful inactivity such as meditation, relaxation or sleep.  Walking is very much a part of their lifestyle and they are constantly engaged in activities such as daily chores which are oftentimes rigorous, walking, gardening, cooking, sight-seeing and appreciating the natural world.  The majority of their time is spent outside.

Centenarians are rarely lonely nor do they stay alone for extended periods of time, however, they do seek their own space. These elders maintain that they have passion and purpose no matter how simple it seems.

To stay alert mentally, centenarians are involved in reading, writing, memorization tasks, joking, singing, music playing, and story-telling.  For example, many of them sing and dance to folk songs, they recite to youngsters their traditions and stories, and they are constantly learning new things.  Sometimes they are simple things such as memorizing special event dates, stories, songs, or poems.

These people identify their traditional healing practices as one of their main foci in the promotion of their health and longevity.  For the most part, these elders do not utilize modern medicine as front-line care, even when it is available.  Traditional healing practices across cultures such as herbalism, granny healers, midwives, Ayurveda, naturopathy, yoga and meditation are resources available to them.  There is a variety of healing practice modalities.  For example, the use of healing plants, thermal equilibrium via "hot" and "cold" plants and foods, quieting the mind through meditation and/or presence, ritual use of the four winds (basically directions) and cosmological and calendrical cycles (based on cycles of our natural world), diverse energies in preparation of medicines and in healing ceremonies, and a multitude of other practices are utilized. As one Maya elder from Belize put it, we conduct our lives "to balance and guide the spirit, giving thanks to the creator and cosmos, the four winds, the four peoples, the four corns, our earth mother."

These traditional elders across cultures live close to nature and have a strong sense of place. Their children grow up learning about herbs and their uses in healing. Kinship networks are strong and families trust and rely on healthcare practices handed down from generations past. Elders are also valued for their wisdom. There is an abiding belief that in most cases medical care begins, and hopefully ends, at home. People also rely on prayer and the power of faith in addressing health problems. To indigenous peoples the environment nurtures health and wellness. Spirit, Mother Earth, and Cosmos are the sources of all medicines and healings. The divisive problems of family, community, and an unhealthful environment invites pathology and deters healing processes. A supportive environment and healthy relationships sustain the individual and enables strength in their healing. Persons need a place they love, a serene place for healing. As a preferred treatment, traditional remedies are utilized, based on one's knowledge that the remedy has worked in the past for self and family members, and oftentimes as a first course of action. When mainstream medical care fails to work, traditional practices, such as herbal medicine, may be successful because traditional practices are in consonance with their culture and employ faith in the spiritual rituals of the healing process.

An interesting custom we found evident across cultures is their daily exercises. Many of these elders and spiritual people awake in the morning at least one hour before sunrise to begin the day. Oftentimes, in India, the elders sun gaze at sunrise and sunset. They do early morning walking, meditation, yoga, which involves stretching or breathing exercises, and cold water bathing among other daily rituals. Their hygiene was uniformly impeccable; oftentimes this meant regular bathing in frigid streams or lakes, steam bathing in natural saunas. And, their oral hygiene is equally impeccable with ritualized regular brushing with teas, herbs, and essential oils; and includes picking, flossing and tongue scraping, and when necessary, nasal and sinus washes with the neti pot to flush out impurities. Yogis are also known to do rectal and colon cleansing in the streams where they live.

Given their passion and purpose, they are oftentimes facilitating constructive development along a variety of fronts. They know who they are and they work to promote self-realization among others. Doing good things for others is paramount to this group of people. Instead of expecting anything in return, they are always eager to assist others, relatives, friends or even strangers. Giving advice and narrating their positive lifestyles to others are part of their daily routines. Since it is part of the traditions to respect elders, their advice is held in high regard. These elders, even if others are not seeking anything, give advice on all types of things such as interpersonal relationships, dietary habits, financial security, and spirituality to name a few. And, a very important practice for these elders is meditation, which brings balance for them and others they guide.

Some of the other characteristic features include: they laugh out loud often, they are very friendly, they behave like children at times, they develop good support networks and extended family members and friends visit them often. There are a high number of well-wishers who surround these elders and in particular the centenarians. These elders have an answer for all questions, whether it is direct or indirect. They insist it comes with their "practice wisdom." They have established a sense of self worth that they work to disseminate.

It is apparent in our study of elderhood, that those who are spiritual contribute to their own peace of mind, their health, and the well-being of their community. There is a consistent "believing in something beyond what you know" among this group. Every day when they awaken, before their meal, before involvement in any auspicious occasions, and before going to sleep, they take a few minutes of their time to give thanks. They are spiritual and oftentimes believe in some form of divinity, also included here as divinity is consciousness. Attributing their secrets of long life to divinity is commonly expressed. They are willing to share their concept of spirituality with others. They are open-minded to others' views. They believe in an afterlife or an after-being of their energy, life force or essence. They allow their intuitions into their consciousness—women seem to express it more. They engage in altered states of consciousness, with fasting, kundalini, meditation and *mantravadam*, music and chanting, and the ingestion of varied beverages and entheogens.

When we examine our modern post-industrial information age society, oftentimes, we have no tradition to guide us on the right path to the Good Life. However, it is there, one must simply dig ones roots, both literally and figuratively. We must find our sense of place in nature and begin to learn, and appreciate once again. Grow our food, revere water and land, nurture our good physiology, mind, spirit and environment, connect to nature, stories, our diverse lineage in our human experience—after all we are all connected. This requires a conscious effort, but is essential to lead a healthy life.

This grounding will continue to assist with ameliorating spurious culture. And, we have so much spurious culture to deal with. Spurious culture includes ideas, values, things, behavior, attitudes, and beliefs that do not satisfy basic needs or physical, mental, and/or spiritual growth. In the modern day, there is a great disposition to buy things to fill a lacuna in the self. It is a materialistic culture with an economy based on consumption of material things, which presages an age of anxiety that corporations exploit in urging people to buy things to make them happy—and the cycle continues. The corporate personality is ruled by the profit motive and the media is the vehicle accessing the consumer. Businesspeople, on whole, generally care little about the health and welfare of the public. The Western ideology of rugged individualism presumes the responsibility of the individual's decision-making. This then becomes the rationale for business to throw anything at the public it can get away with, rationalizing that the individual should make their own purchasing decisions. Because of media-hype, making choices for healthier lifestyles has become a difficult task for the uninformed citizen. Add this to the fact that self-realization and informed decision-making require a special education and cultivation and are essentially art forms that improve with practice. The challenge for those of us who promote a healthy lifestyle and a healthy society is fighting to neutralize toxic information that originates from the ruling corporate elite. A viable health promotion paradigm requires education at all levels of society, beginning with parental influence and control. Becoming conscious of what poisons deteriorate our quality of life is a paramount objective in achieving quality of life for all.

In sum: what do we learn from the teachers-elders of traditional society? They show that with a relatively comprehensive, but simple set of practices we can enhance our vitality and promote longevity. They demonstrate the importance of a positive mental outlook. They show the importance and ease obtaining balance through holistic living with deep regard and respect for nature and all its life forms. They demonstrate the importance of stress minimization. They love and teach a respect for and appreciation of the cycles of life and the events of the life course and our connections to the natural world in these cycles. They illustrate the need for consistent physical and mental exercise, and the need for time spent outside and in nature. They teach that we must learn of our passion and purpose no matter how insignificant it is to others. They lead by example in demonstrating that we must care for and respect one another. And, that we must teach our children these important ways. Through their dietary and nutritional practices, they show that most of our disease burdens could be resolved through clean, natural water consumption (for this we need intact areas of ecological integrity) and diets rich in plants and whole foods and with a minimum of animal products and absolutely no processed foods. In short, we thrive on calorie sparse, nutrient dense, plant-based foods.

In this era of genetic testing, telemedicine, incredibly high priced pharmaceutical drugs, and expensive invasive medical procedures to extend the life of people is largely unwarranted and unsuccessful as illustrated by decreasing life expectancy of late. With limited resources and unlimited needs, these practices are unsustainable and largely unnecessary.

On an institutional level, government must support and enforce an ecology that maintains a healthy, sustainable environment and encourages a balance of nature, cares for the people while frustrating the narcissism and greed of the oligarchy. This involves community leaders who are knowledgeable about the healthy living of humans, animals and plant life and serve the principles of the balance of nature and who maintain the priority of ecology over the convenience of jobs.

Government must promote educational institutions whose members teach healthy living, promote mind-building mentalities, including music and dance, creative expression, recreation and creativity of individual students; where school food-places serve items that help brains grow and eliminate those items that contribute to the mental and social ills of youth, *viz.*, sugar, fat, preservatives, hydrogenated oils, and caffeine. On this same governmental level we must expand our federally-funded parent agencies that provide information for informed living and healthy childrearing. On this institutional level members of religious institutions must teach the qualities of spirituality and appreciate the balance of powers of the universe.

On the level of individual well-being there must be a sense of mission and calling, vision and commitment. One's work must excite with the expectation of fulfillment.

One can create an identity around a mission in one's life. Satellite activities in life should be built around and be in conjunction with the mission. Other parameters of spirituality and wellbeing include the following:

**Nutrition.** Know the foods and supplements that promote health and wellness. These include the phytochemicals including plant sterols and phytoestrogens, plant pigments like anthocyanins and carotenoids, antioxidants, vitamins and minerals like Vitamin D, calcium and magnesium, immune enhancers, herbs and spices, and clean water, and many other food supplements for specific organ functions. It is common knowledge today that the major detriments to health and vitality include excessive caffeine, sugar, fat, hydrogenated oils, preservatives and chemicals in foods, alcohol, and nicotine. A nutrient-rich, calorie sparse plant based diet is key. And, eat organic! Do not put toxic chemicals into your body.

**Hygiene.** Cleanliness involves all body/mind systems: skin, hair, nails, sinuses, lungs, alimentary canal from mouth to anus, organs, including the brain and the thoughts, images, and feelings of the mind-body.

**Exercise.** This includes aerobic activity for the cardiovascular system, physical resistance work for adequate stress of muscle on bone, stretching to loosen joints and tendons and disperse stress—yoga is one of the best disciplines for this; pubococcygeus work to maintain a powerful pelvic floor and sexual vitality, breathing and meditation exercises complete this list.

**Psychosocial vitality.** Maintain a positive attitude, avoid fatalistic thinking, see barriers to goals or problems as challenges rather than threats, maintain self-reliance, cultivate introspection through meditation, and see each individual encountered as a world exciting to explore.

**Social involvement.** Engage in community activities and issues; create sources of community support. Create relationships of intimacy among same-sex peers sharing a common mission and psychosocial reinforcement. Create relationships of intimacy with opposite sex peers, sharing mutual needs and concerns; and maintain an active sexual relationship for bonding and support.

**Education.** Consider the learning experience as a never-ending goal in life. Develop continuous, on-going learning goals toward higher levels of consciousness. Realms of learning include the areas of intellectual pursuit, music, kinesthetic development, art, language-learning and poetry, arts and crafts, travel and ethnographic experience, teaching, spiritual perspectives—including spiritual and/or religious ideology and eastern spirituality such as yoga.

**The Spiritual Quest.** Practice yoga, chi gung, tai chi, and other meditative disciplines. Develop a spiritual quest through one's adopted spiritual cosmology and evolve a transcendental perspective and life practice. Connect to nature and dig your roots. Respect our elders and our environment—pass this along! In essence, cultivate consciousness.

The authors learn directly from traditional, longest-living peoples who live in the Great Lakes region and Appalachian Mountains of North America; Maya Mountains of Belize, Central America; Amazonia and Andean highlands of Peru, South America; Western Ghats of Kerala and Tamil Nadu, India, and extending into Sri Lanka; and Afromontane and Albertine rift regions of Ethiopia. There are long-lived elders among many cultures the world over. Our findings closely mirror those in these various diverse cultures including the Mediterranean region, the high valleys of the Himalayas, the Caucasus Mountains, and in Okinawa; [8] they live healthy lifestyles by following tradition and taking care of body, mind, spirit and the environment within which they reside. The knowledge of right living is present perhaps given the remote nature of these pristine places. [9] We must preserve the ecological integrity and biodiversity upon which we all depend. We must engage our universities, our hospitals, our industries, our students, and our children and position them to act to attenuate the pollution that degrades our quality of life.

# Notes

## Chapter 1 Notes

1. Chopra, D. (2000). Holistic Revolution. London: Allen Lane.
2. Charaka Samhita — Sharma PV (translator) (1981). Chaukhamba Orientalia, Varanasi, India, pp. ix-xxxii (I) 4 Volumes.
3. Valiathan, M.S. (2003). The Legacy of Caraka. Chennai, India: Longman.
4. Alphen, J.V.and Aris, A. (1997). Oriental Medicine: An Illustrated Guide to the Ancient Arts of Healing. London: Serindia Publications.
5. Woodham, A. and Peters, D. (2004). Encyclopedia of Healing Therapies. New York: Dorling Kindersley.
6. Murray, M. and Pizzorno, J. (2003). Encyclopedia of Natural Medicine. Rocklin, CA: Prime Publishing.
7. Concato, J., Shah, N., and, Horwitz, R. (2000). Randomized, Controlled Trials, Observational Studies, and the Hierarchy of Research Designs. N Engl J Med: 342:1887-92.
8. Farnsworth, N., Akerele, O., Bingel, A., Soejarto, D., and Guo, Z., (1985). Medicinal Plants in Therapy. Bulletin of the World Health Organization, 63(6):965-981.
9. World Health Organization (2002). WHO Traditional Medicine Strategy 2002-2005. Geneva, Switzerland (WHO/EDM/TRM/2002.1).
10. Eisenberg DM, Davis RB, Ettner SL, Appel S, Wilkey S, Van Rompay M, et al. (1998). Trends in alternative medicine use in the United States, 1990-1997: Results of a follow-up national survey. JAMA: 280: 1569-1575.
11. Barnes PM, Bloom B, Nahin R. (2008). CDC National Health Statistics Report #12. Complementary and Alternative Medicine Use Among Adults and Children: United States, 2007.
12. Pesek, T., Helton, L. R., & Nair, M. (2006). Healing across cultures: Learning from traditions. EcoHealth. 3(2): 114-118.
13. French, S. and Rogers, G. (2004). A First Look at New LOHAS Consumer Research. LOHAS Journal's Factbook. 5(1) 26-28 and 66-67.

## Chapter 2 Notes

1. DeGrasse Tyson, N., and Goldsmith, D. (2004). *Origins: Fourteen billion years of cosmic evolution.* W. W. Norton & Company, New York
2. Chartrand, M. (1991). *National Audubon Society: Field guide to the night sky.* Alfred A. Knopf, New York
3. Hennacy Powell, D. (2009). *The ESP Enigma: The Scientific Case for Psychic Phenomina*, Walker Publishing Company, New York

4.  Raven, P., Evert, R., and Eichhorn, S. (2005). *Biology of Plants.* W.H. Freeman and Company, New York

5.  Fortey, R. (1997). *Life: A Natural History of the First Four Billion Years of Life on Earth.* Random House, New York.

6.  Davis, W. (2009). The Wayfinders: Why Ancient Wisdom Matters in the Modern World. House of Anansi Press, Toronto, ON.

7.  Deitsch, R., Lonky, S. (2007). Invisible Killers: The Truth About Environmental Genocide, I.K. Enterprises, Inc.

8.  Pesek T, Helton L, and Nair M. (2006). Healing across cultures: Learning from traditions. *EcoHealth Journal*; 3(2):114-118.

9.  Maffi L., editor. *On Biological and Cultural Diversity*, Smithsonian Institution Press, Washington and London, UK; (2001).

10. Sutherland, W. Parallel extinction risk and global distribution of languages and species. *Nature*. (2003); 423: 276-279.

11. Davis, W. (1999). *Clouded Leopard.* Douglas and MacIntyre Publishing Group, Vancouver, BC.

12. Grimes, B. (1996). *Ethnologue: Languages of the World.* 13th Ed. Dallas: Summer Institute of Linguistics.

13. United Nations Food and Agricultural Organization. (2000). *Global forest resources assessment.* Available at: http://www.fao.org/forestry/fo/fra/main/ (FAO Forestry Paper 140. United Nations). Accessed August 3, 2005.

14. WWF. *Living Planet Report 2004.* Gland, Switzerland: World Wildlife Fund; (2004).

15. Hanski, I. (2005). Landscape fragmentation, biodiversity loss and the societal response. *EMBO Reports*; 6(5): 388-392.

16. Stepp J, Castaneda H, Cervone S. (2005). Mountains and biocultural diversity. *Mountain Research and Development*. 25(3):223-227.

17. Hayden, C. (2003). *When Nature Goes Public: The Making and Unmaking of Bioprospecting in Mexico.* Princeton University Press, Princeton, NJ.

18. Berlin, B. and Berlin, E. (2003). *NGO's and the process of prior informed consent in bioprospecting research: the Maya ICBG project in Chiapas, Mexico.* UNESCO, Blackwell Publishing Ltd, Oxford, UK.

19. Nigh, R. (2002). Maya Medicine in the Biological Gaze. *Current Anthropology*. 43(3): 451-477.

20. Alexiades, M. (2004). Ethnobiology and Globalization: Science and Ethics at the turn of the Century. in Carlson, J. and Maffi, L. editors. *Ethnobotany and Conservation of Biocultural Diversity.* Advances in Economic Botany, 15. The New York Botanical Garden Press. New York.

21. Bannister, K. and Barrett, K. (2004). Weighing the Proverbial "Ounce of Prevention" against the "Pound of Cure" in a Biocultural Context: A Role for the Precautionary Principle in Ethnobiological Research. in Carlson, J. and Maffi, L, editors. *Ethnobotany and Conservation of Biocultural Diversity.* Advances in Economic Botany, 15. The New York Botanical Garden Press. New York.
22. Pesek, T., Cal, V., Fini, N., Cal, M., Rojas, M., Sanchez, P., Poveda, L., Collins, S., Knight, K., Arnason, J. (2007). Itzama: Revival of Traditional Healing by the Q'eqchi' Maya of Southern Belize. *HerbalGram.* 76:34-43.
23. Atran, S. (1993). Itza Maya Tropical Agro-Forestry. *Current Anthropology.* 34(5): 633-700.
24. Kashanipour, R., McGee, R.J. (2004). Northern Lacandon Maya Medicinal Plant Use in the Communities of Lacanja Chan Sayab and Naha', Chiapas, Mexico. *Journal of Ecological Anthropology.* 8:47-66.
25. Barrera-Bassols, N., Toledo, V. (2005). Ethnoecology of the Yucatec Maya: Symbolism, Knowledge, and Management of Natural Resources. *Journal of Latin American Geography.* 4(1): 9-41.
26. Treyvaud-Amiguet, V., Arnason, J., Maquin, P., Cal, V., Sanchez-Vindaz, P., and Poveda, L. (2005). A Consensus Ethnobotany of the Q'eqchi' Maya of Southern Belize. *Economic Botany.* 59(1): 29-42.

**Chapter 3 Notes**
1. Guyton and Hall. (2006). Textbook of Medical Physiology. 11th Edition. Elsevier, Philadelphia, Pennsylvania.
2. Valtin and Schafer. (1995). Renal Function. 3rd Edition. Lippincott, Williams, and Wilkins, New York.
3. Environmental Working Group. (2005). *Body Burdon – The pollution in newborns.* Retrieved 05/22/2010 from: http://www.ewg.org/reports/bodyburden2/execsumm.php
4. Experimental Man. (2010). Main Page. Retrieved 05/22/2010 from: http://www.experimentalman.com/
5. Johson, M., Kenney, N., Stoica, A., Hilakivi-Clarke, L., Singh, B., Chepko, G., Clarke, R., Sholler, P., Lirio, A., Foss, C., Reiter, R., Trock, B., Paik, S., & Martin, M.B., (2003). Cadmium mimics the effects of estrogens *in vivo* in the uterus and mammary gland. *Nat. Med.* 9, 1081-1084.
6. Colborn, T., Vom Saal, F.S. & Soto, A.M. (1993). Developmental effects of endocrine-disrupting chemicals in wildlife and humans. *Environ. Health Perspect.* 101, 378-384.
7. Safe, S. (2000). Endocrine distruptors and human health - is there a problem: an update. *Environ. Health Perspect.* 108, 487-493.

8. Martin, M.B., Reiter, R., Pham, T., Avellanet, Y., Camara, J., Lahm, M., Pentecost, E., Pratap, K., Gilmore, B., Divekar, S., Dagata, R., Bull, J., Stoica, A. (2003). Estrogen-like activity of metals in MCF-7 breast cancer cells. *Endocrinology* 144, 2425-2436.

9. Goyer, R.A. (1986). Toxic effects of metals. in *Toxic Effects of Metals in Toxicology: The Basic Science of Poisons* 3rd edn. (eds. Klassen, C.D., Andur, M.D. & Doull, J.) 582-635, MacMillan, New York.

10. World Health Organization. (2002). *WHO Traditional Medicine Strategy 2002-2005.* Geneva, Switzerland: World Health Organization.

11. Farnsworth, N., Akerele, O., Bingel, A., Soejarto, D., and Guo, Z. (1985). Medicinal Plants in Therapy. *Bulletin of the World Health Organization,* 63(6):965-981.

12. Willett, W.C. (2002). Balancing life-style and genomics research for disease prevention. *Science* 296:695-698.

13. Emerson-Lombardo, N.B. (2008). Responding to Early-Stage Alzheimer's Using an Innovative Nutrition Program. *Dimensions.* 15(1).

14. Davis CD, Hartmuller V, Freedman M, Hartge P, Picciano MF, Swanson CA, Milner JA. (2007). Vitamin D and cancer: current dilemmas and future needs. Nutr Rev. 65:S71-S74.

15. Hyppönen E, Läärä E, Reunanen A, Järvelin MR, Virtanen SM. (2001). Intake of vitamin D and risk of type 1 diabetes: a birth-cohort study. *Lancet.* 358:1500-3.

16. Pittas AG, Dawson-Hughes B, Li T, Van Dam RM, Willett WC, Manson JE, et al. (2006). Vitamin D and calcium intake in relation to type 2 diabetes in women. *Diabetes Care.* 29:650-6.

17. Krause R, Bühring M, Hopfenmüller W, Holick MF, Sharma AM. (1998). Ultraviolet B and blood pressure. *Lancet.* 352:709-10.

18. Hicks, G.E., Shardell, M., Miller, R.R., et al. (2008). Associations Between Vitamin D Status and Pain in Older Adults: The Invecchiare in Chianti Study. *Journal of the American Geriatrics Society,* 56(5), 785-791.

19. Munger KL, Levin LI, Hollis BW, Howard NS, Ascherio A. (2006). Serum 25-hydroxyvitamin D levels and risk of multiple sclerosis. *JAMA.* 296:2832-8.

20. Van den Berg H. (1997). Bioavailability of vitamin D. *Eur J Clin Nutr.* 51:S76-9.

21. Holick MF. (2003). Evolution and function of vitamin D. Recent results. *Cancer Res.* 164:3-28.

22. Hayes CE, Hashold FE, Spach KM, Pederson LB. (2003). The immunological functions of the vitamin D endocrine system. *Cell Mol Biol.* 49:277-300.

23. Cranney C, Horsely T, O'Donnell S, Weiler H, Ooi D, Atkinson S, et al. (2007). Effectiveness and safety of vitamin D. *AHRQ Publication No. 07-E013*. Rockville, MD: Agency for Healthcare Research and Quality.

24. Wolpowitz D, Gilchrest BA. (2006). The Vitamin D questions: How much do you need and how should you get it? *J Am Acad Dermatol*. 54:301-17.

25. Holick MF, MacLaughlin JA, Clark MB, Holick SB, Potts JT Jr, Anderson RR, et al. (1980). Photosynthesis of previtamin D3 in human skin and the physiologic consequences. *Science*. 210(4466):203-5.

26. Deitsch, R., Lonky, S. (2007). Invisible Killers, The truth about environmental genocide. Invisible Killer Enterprises.

**Chapter 4 Notes**

1. Nussbaum, P. (2007). *Your Brain Health Lifestyle*. Word Association Publishers.

2. Hanson, R. (2009). *Buddha's Brain*. New Harbinger Publications.

3. Sylvia, C. (1997). *Change of Heart*. Little Brown.

4. Powell, D.H. (2009). *The ESP Enigma: The Scientific Case for Psychic Phenomina*, Walker Publishing Company.

5. Allgire, K. (2010). The Five Vrttis: Fluctuations of Consciousness. *Balanced Living Magazine*, Winter.

6. Kabat-Zinn, J. (1990). *Full Catastrophe Living: Using the Wisdom of Your Body and Mind to Face Stress, Pain, and Illness*. Dell Publishing.

7. Austin, J. H. (1998). *Zen and the Brain*. The MIT Press.

8. Barnes, V. (2003). Impact of stress reduction on negative school behavior in adolescents. *Health and Quality of Life Outcomes. 1(1)*.

9. Winzelberg, A., Luskin, F. (1999). "The effect of meditation training in stress levels in secondary school teachers." *Stress Medicine*. 15: 69-77.

10. Shannahoff-Khalsa, D. (2003). "Kundalini Yoga Meditation Techniques for the Treatment of Obsessive-Compulsive & OC Spectrum Disorders" *Brief Treatment and Crisis Intervention*. 3: 369-382.

11. Collins, Michael P., Dunn, Lucia F. (2005) "The Effects of Meditation and Visual Imagery on an Immune System Disorder: Dermatomyositis." *Journal of Alternative & Complementary Medicine 11(2)*: 275.

12. Afari, N., Eisenberg, D. (2000). "Use of alternative treatments by chronic fatigue syndrome discordant twins." *Integrative Medicine. 2(2)*: 97-103.

13. Tedlock, B. (2005). *The Woman in the Shaman's Body*. Bantom Books.

14. Rubel, W., Arora, D. (2008). A Study of Cultural Bias in Field Guide Determinations of Mushroom Edibility Using the Iconic Mushroom, Amanita muscaria, as an Example. Economic Botany, 62(3).

## Chapter 5 Notes

1. Random House College Dictionary. (1995). 1290.
2. Dictionary.com (2010). Available at: http://dictionary.reference.com/browse/spirit (Dictionary.com main page). Accessed May 26, 2010.
3. Hennacy Powell, D. (2009). *The ESP Enigma: The Scientific Case for Psychic Phenomina*, Walker Publishing Company, New York.
4. Moro P, Myers J, Lehmann A. (2008). *Magic, Witchcraft, and Religion*, 7th ed., McGraw Hill Publishers.
5. Federal Interagency Forum on Aging-Related Statistics (FIFARS). (2008). Older Americans 2008: Key Indicators of Well-Being. Federal Interagency Forum on Aging-Related Statistics, Washington, DC: U.S. Government Printing Office.
6. De Ropp, R. (2008). Psychedelic Drugs and Religious Experience. In *Magic, Witchcraft, and Religion*. Moro, Myers, and Lehmann. 7th ed., McGraw Hill Publishers.
7. Foster, R., and Hicks, G. (1999). *How We Choose to be Happy*. Putnam.
8. Reminick, R. (1988). *Black Ethnicity: A Conceptualization of Black Culture, Social Organization, and Personality*. Kendall Hunt Publishers.
9. Aberle, D. (1965). A Note on Relative Deprivation Theory as Applied to Millenarian and Other Cult Movements. In *Reader in Comparative Religion: An Anthropological Approach*. Lessa and Vogt, 2nd ed.
10. Wallace, A.F.C. (1956). Revitalization Movements. *American Anthropologist*. 58:264-281.
11. Parenti, M. (1964). The Black Muslims: From Revolution to Institution. *Social Research*. 31:175-194.
12. Ray, P., and Anderson, S.R. (2000). *The Cultural Creatives*. Harmony Books, New York.
13. Conscious Wave. (2008). *LOHAS Online*. Available at: http://www.lohas.com/about.html Retrieved May 27, 2010.

## Chapter 6 Notes

1. World Health Organization. (1946). Constitution of the World Health Organization, Geneva, 1946.
2. Pesek, T., Helton, L., and Nair, M. (2006). Healing Across Cultures: Learning from Traditions. *EcoHealth*. 3(2).
3. Pesek, T., Cal, V., Fini, N., Cal, M., Rojas, M., Sanchez, P., Poveda, L., Collins, S., Knight, K., Arnason, J. (2007). Itzama: Revival of Traditional Healing by the Q'eqchi' Maya of Southern Belize. *HerbalGram*. 76:34-43.

4. Pesek T., Helton L., Reminick R., D. Kannan, Nair M. (2008). "Healing Traditions of Southern India and the Conservation of Culture and Biodiversity: A Preliminary Study" *Ethnobotany Research and Applications*. 6: 471-479.

5. Pesek T., Abramiuk, M., Garagic, D., Fini, N., Meerman, J., Cal, V. (2009). Sustaining Plants and People: Traditional Q'eqchi' Maya Botanical Knowledge and Interactive Spatial Modeling in Prioritizing Conservation of Medicinal Plants for Culturally Relative Holistic Health Promotion *EcoHealth*. 6(1): 79-90.

6. Pesek T., Abramiuk M., Cal V., Rojas M., Collins S., Sanchez P., Poveda L., Arnason, J. (2010). Q'eqchi' Maya Healers Traditional Knowledge in Prioritizing Conservation of Medicinal Plants: Culturally Relative Conservation in Sustaining Traditional Holistic Health Promotion. *Biodiversity and Conservation*. 19(1): 1-20.

7. Federal Interagency Forum on Aging-Related Statistics (FIFARS). (2008). Older Americans 2008: Key Indicators of Well-Being. Federal Interagency Forum on Aging-Related Statistics, Washington, DC: U.S. Government Printing Office.

8. Robbins J. (2007). Healthy at 100. Ballantine Books, The Random House Publishing Group.

9. Stepp J., Castaneda H., Cervone S. (2005). Mountains and biocultural diversity. *Mountain Research and Development*. 25(3):223-227.